I0545688

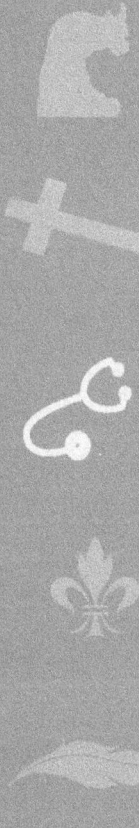

The Evolve Fertility Series

by Beth Alderman, MD, MPH

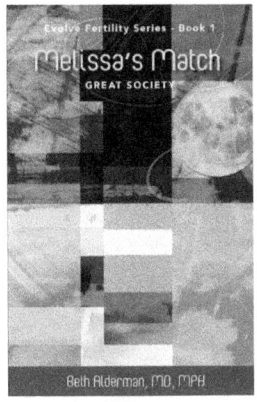

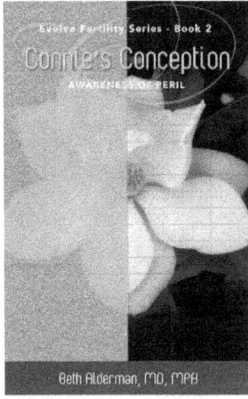

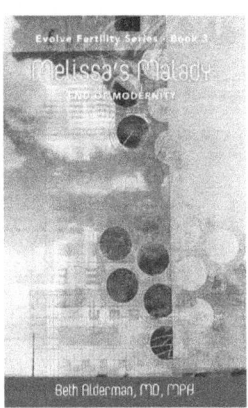

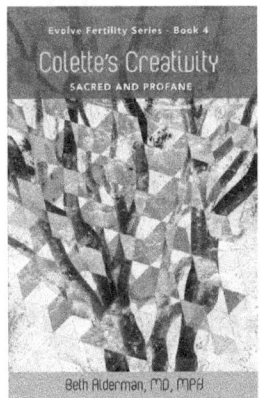

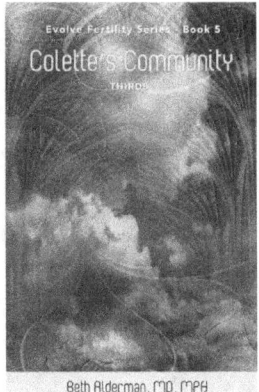

Melissa's Malady

END OF MODERNITY

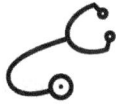

Book Three of the
Evolve Fertility Series

Beth Alderman, MD, MPH

LIVING FUTURE BOOKS • ASHLAND, OREGON

Melissa's Malady: End of Modernity
by Beth Alderman, MD, MPH
© 2019 FutureMedicine, LLC
www.LivingFutureBooks.com

For related online courses visit
www.LivingFutureCourses.com

All rights reserved. No part of this book may be used or reproduced
by any means without the written permission of the author except
in the case of brief quotations embodied in critical
articles and reviews.

Editor: Julie Clayton
Cover Art: BruceBayard.com
Book Design: BookSavvyStudio.com

Library of Congress Control Number: 2019903850
ISBN: 978-1-7321110-2-8
First Edition
Printed in the United States of America

Contents

To Anna

*Today, the canals of Leiden are clean, models
of the modern Dutch commitment to water
quality, but... in the early seventeenth century,
at the behest of the dominant, expansion-minded
textile barons, officials began to install brick sewer
infrastructure that was much cheaper to maintain
than cesspits. Though this period concides with the
prosperous era known as the "Dutch Golden Age,"
public health in Leiden fell off steeply.*

— WILL HUNT

1

Care

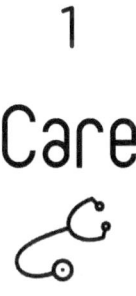

John taps the crystal of his watch. Melissa is three minutes late already. He descends the steps of the Hutchinson Commons to look south along the gray stone wall of the quadrangle of the University of Chicago. Below a line of gargoyles that stare fiercely out at nothing, a gray-haired man in a bowtie is lugging an overfilled shoulder bag toward the grassy stripe of the sunken Midway at 59th Street. John sighs tensely. At the office he could have used those three minutes to make a call, or to send an email. He could have removed an item from his interminable to-do list.

"John?"

The timbre of her voice stops his breath. When he turns he is shocked to see her unmistakable pale blue eyes bracketed by creases and topped by a fringe of fading hair. She is no longer the fresh-faced idealist who awakened his manhood. His sexual fantasies fade. *What am I doing here?*

Melissa's lips resist a smile.

John extends his hand and says too heartily, "Missy, good to see you!"

She gives his hand a quick shake. She seems cool, wary even. They walk west on 57th Street. John starts toward the science buildings in the distance. They represent leaps in modern design, but look to him like upended shoeboxes. As she falls in step, he says, "Not much has changed here."

"Hmmm."

"My sister says hello."

"Ah."

"Hot for September, isn't it?"

"Mmm-hmm."

He tosses a few more conversational balls. She lets them drop. He begins to feel uneasy until it occurs to him that she is probably staying silent to gain the advantage. In a meeting, everyone turns to the silent one. John steals a glance at her face to calculate her next move and is surprised to find her looking at him expectantly. *What does she want?* The inquiry caroms through his neural nets like a bit traveling the Internet and dissolves into anxiety. He feels damp circles spreading under his armpits. The silence between them thickens like taffy.

Melissa shakes her head lightly and enters the graceful wrought iron gates that lead to the quadrangle's courtyards. As John follows, he is lifted by a wave of nostalgia. It was here that he lived the ponderous Life of the Mind, which freed him from the unexamined life, and revealed to him the perils integral to the power of reason. He remembers the heady joy of delving deeply into wonder, struggling with problems that forced him to face the unknown, and to expand the boundaries of his inner world. He remembers that these ascetic pleasures could be erotic, and once bound him to her.

"Do you have anything to say to me?" she asks pointedly.

He turns to see that she has stopped and is staring at him. A knot of concern rises between her brows. His eyes fix on her forehead, which expresses something he cannot read. Finally, she asks him, "Do you you remember that the last time we talked you said you were going to come and visit me in Oregon?"

"When was that?"

"Before you disappeared from my life and stopped responding to my calls. That was 1977. This is 1997."

"We spoke then, didn't we? Broke up?"

"Just so you know, I intend to hold you responsible for everything that you do—and everything that you don't." She turns and walks on.

John follows Melissa through a walkway lit by leaded-glass windows, dipping his head to avoid the low-peaked doorway. The walkway's small scale reminds him that the quadrangle is a copy of Cambridge College in England, and that like its medieval model, its cold stones bear the marks of artisans' hands. When they emerge into a courtyard, John takes a deep breath and looks up at the lacy elms, which appear lush in the golden sunlight of fall.

John hears the echo of thudding footsteps and turns to see Melissa racing up the stairs of a brown-painted temporary theater. She hops onto the wide wooden stage, raises her face to the dappled shade, and spins like a little girl. She halts, off-balance, laughing. "Remember the Shakespeare plays?"

John shakes his head. His memory is like the walls of their old bedroom, which were covered by layers and layers of paper and paint. His childhood, college, and medical school years are covered up with years of success on success. He is glad that medical school, which was a blur of late night vigils over stuporous drunks and manipulative drug-addicts, is long forgotten.

"You must remember Professor Pratt! He looked like a huge pincushion in his Pierrot collar and puffy bloomers! And he would always forget his lines when he tried to be funny! You used to stuff towels in your trousers and mimic him!"

John remembers being a skinny, beret-wearing boy, but doesn't recall being so sophomoric. He regrets the inanity of her memories until she smiles and the spark in her eyes ignites something in his heart, and the old electricity courses between them. The intensity of this timeless vital connection topples the idol of material success. He had dismissed his love for her as a passing neurochemical phenomenon, and his persistent interest as part of a prevailing cultural pattern like pining for the past, seeking escape, or trying to smash repression with transgression.

Now that he feels their living connection he recognizes it as a source of meaning and purpose. He doesn't know what it is, but that doesn't bother him. He is used to recognizing things by matching their patterns to the ones he has been storing in his mind. He is also used to rationalizing them. He tells himself that she is the best friend he ever had, the one who sees him as he is and can witness his life and give him advice. He has had no one to confide in, until now.

When she leaves the courtyard and leads him to the traffic circle at the heart of the quad, she looks back to make sure he is keeping up. This sweet solicitude fills him with the feeling that he has always been with her and will be safe in her even when she is gone. It also worries him. She once bounded ahead on the road of life without looking back at him. He wants her to feel that way again. He wants her to trust him. How foolish he was to stay when she left for Oregon. He lacked the confidence then to know that he could succeed anywhere.

Melissa stops in the shade of a large maple near a neatly tended bed of red geraniums and turns to look into his eyes again. "So, how have things turned out for you?"

He is always ready for that question. He pulls up his broad shoulders, glad he worked to stay in shape, and leans easily against the rough bark of the maple trunk to rattle off the career moves that are his trump card in every game he plays with superiors, peers, and subordinates. Half way through his recited résumé, though, the words catch in his throat. She is disappointed. He rushes to finish up, exaggerating his role in national advisory groups, and emphasizing his early promotion to Chair of the Department of Medicine at Northwestern University Medical School.

To buy time, he asks her the same question, and is flummoxed by her answer. She works part-time as a hospitalist in Denver, which means she has a dead-end job that is so far down the hierarchy as to be outside it. More astonishing, she isn't embarrassed to admit it, which must mean that his success does not impress her. He feels angry at her obtuseness, and then accepts her judgment. No vaccine, disease, or treatment bears his name. He should have worked harder. He should have tried for the Nobel Prize and left the passing needs of the dying to others.

John squelches his omnipresent need to do more, and his resultant sense of inadequacy. He knows how to rally. The machinery of modernity has been hurling pitches at him for years in the batting cage of life. When he sees one coming he swings dutifully, hits it into the net, and tells himself it's a homer. His mentors used to tell him, but now he does this for himself and others. When he cannot deny a miss, he resolves never to miss again. This habit makes it is easy to believe he will prevail every day, including today, the day he blocked out on his calendar to lure Melissa back into his life. He'll have to play his cards right. He doesn't want to risk their friendship.

She has already moved on. He follows toward a small court-yard south of the traffic circle and stops there by her side. They are facing an abstract bronze statue, the pedestal of which bears the title "Why?" It reaches up toward sky like a questioning hand.

Melissa laughs. "Remember graduation, when you taped a sign on it that said, 'Why not?'"

For the first time in a long time, John feels his face light up. "Yes! But I didn't tape it to the statue. I put it on a bulldozer sitting over there." He points to the lawn beside the tennis courts. "And we sat over there," he points across the quadrangle to the stairs of Eckhart Hall, "and watched people react. I never got so many laughs from strangers!"

"Oh, I don't know. You got quite a few at those Black Student Organization dances." She smiles slyly. She, too, is feeling easier.

"I think they were trying not to laugh at either of us." John grins buoyantly. He searches her face for answers. To his surprise, he finds one.

I remember who I was then! A funny and creative guy immersed in friends and music. When he has fallen into step with her, and is sharing with her a haphazard list of reminiscences, John realizes with a rush of gratification that she is returning his stories to him. *This is it! This is the reason I came! You are the witness to my life. I want to tell you everything.*

They wend back around to the corner where they met earlier. Melissa stands on the edge of the curb and looks caddy-corner to the Unitarian Church and its Blue Gargoyle Café, where they used to eat lunch. She scoops a strand of hair behind her ear. The gesture transports him back to the days when they walked this way to class.

To avoid a quagmire of complex feelings he points to the Blue

Gargoyle and says as lightly as he can, "Remember when eating whole grain bread was a radical act?"

"I remember the set you played in that sanctuary." When he doesn't reply, she pursues pointedly, "You do remember, don't you?"

John opens his mouth to say yes, but shakes his head no.

"Well, you played brilliantly, as usual. I could have listened forever. We knew so many extraordinary kids then!"

"Like yourself."

"Oh geez, John. Since when did you get to be full of it?"

"You still can't take a compliment."

She laughs. "Touché! I'm still the Scandinavian girl from Peoria. But what about you? Back then you were confident without being stuck up or artificial. I loved that—liked that in you."

"A lot of water under the bridge."

As they walk, a silence enfolds them like the peace of a perfect dawn that would be exalted by bird song but broken by words. In their delicate recesses, their hearts reweave the web that once joined them, and their feelings try and trust the strands' integrity. Her wariness eases, and he forgets that he once wanted to win.

When John speaks again his tone is warm. "I'm due for a sabbatical soon."

"How wonderful! Tell me all about it!"

He talks of going to France for the summer. They trade tales of places they have visited, lingering on the pleasures of cuisine, culture, and nature. When she describes a visit to Rome, John pictures them lying in bed together in the afternoon, the sun's rays warming their naked skins. He can almost feel the warm breeze that wafts over them, bringing the aroma of eggplant in olive oil.

As they reminisce, John's mind is a one-man play. He wants

Melissa to know everything, but wants her to see it his way. While he is speaking his truth as best he can, his subconscious mind is backstage juggling the logistics of linking the past and the future. Each of these irreconcilable nothings carries so much weight in his mind that he will, sooner or later, have to drop one and dive for the other. In the meantime, the play is distracting him from his tragic mask, which is hidden beneath a mask of success, and his comic mask, which is gathering dust in a prop room.

By the time they pass by Blackwood Avenue and take a slight detour to peer into the lobby of Blackwood Hall, they are talking easily, and have worked out an impromptu language rich in medical phrases and in slang from their college years. Farther along at Powell's Bookstore, when John glimpses their reflection against the shop fronts across the street, past and present merge in his mind and he is able to imagine that they were never apart.

John has no interest in the bookstore. He hasn't read for pleasure in years and isn't about to start. He watches impatiently as Melissa runs her fingers over the spines of books that are lined up on a pinewood stand outside the entrance. When she enters, he follows, and uses the time to make a circuit of the floor-to-ceiling shelves, which are still crammed with books on an astonishing array of subjects. He stops in the brightly lit reading area in the center, which is new since his last visit, and is furnished with chairs and display tables. Melissa gathers a few volumes and sits down to peruse them.

John goes outside to wait. He passes time by observing the street, which is busy with locals who are out and about on this beautiful Saturday afternoon. He peruses passing cars and eavesdrops on pedestrians. He picks up threads of conversation that reveal the warp and weft of a living community. In a moment of strange stillness, John realizes that he knew only a small part of Hyde Park in his youth and recalls less.

His mask of success slips. He can see now that fear of failure misled him. He should not try for the Nobel. He already spends far too much time at work. Over the years his schedule inflated like the consumer economy that is eating up more and more of his income, and became as bloated as his patients who eat more and more and more. If he had left Hyde Park as planned, he would have a happy home with the love of his life instead of a crushing routine of thankless striving that leaves no room for his heart's desires.

When Melissa emerges from the store cradling a new book, something about talking with teenagers, they head north toward the commercial strip on 53rd Street. He resumes their conversation by saying, "Look, I know you don't think much of my status."

"John, I didn't say—"

"Don't deny it. I don't either. I just want to tell you about my pet projects, things I've been able to do because the Dean has to keep me happy."

John improvises a hasty résumé of good works. He tells her that between battles for space, money, and prestige, he started a program that enabled freshman medical students to visit patients in homes and hospices. There they could see patients in the context of their lives, which would humanize their care in a way that would be impossible in a hospital or clinic. He co-founded a program that offers inner city students summer jobs in his laboratories and clinics. He created an alumni network to help keep rural graduates up to date. These secret successes are the source of his soul pride. He sneaks a sideways glance at Melissa's face and is relieved and pleased to see that she approves.

After a pause she laughs. "I admire that, I really do, but after seven e-mails and two hours of face time, you still haven't acknowledged that you did me wrong."

"I didn't measure up. I'm not proud of it. I didn't mention it because I thought you wouldn't see me."

"I'm sorry, did you just apologize? I must have missed it."

"I'm sorry. I am. Sorry. I, uh—"

"Do me a favor and cut the crap."

He opens his mouth but snaps it shut when he realizes she is right. Right up until he saw that she was disappointed by his achievements, he assumed that she would automatically agree that his successes justified his abandoning her. She doesn't see it that way and won't let him rationalize his behavior. She eschews pretense and won't let him get away with anything. Unexpectedly, a long-buried part of John's psyche feels loved.

I must free her from this for good. He resolves to protect her from this and every other threat, including, if need be, the agenda of his desires.

They head north and past the crabgrass-infested turf of a playground at the west edge of a pocket park. Fractious preschoolers in various states of misery and delight are taking turns jumping onto a pile of wood chips under the watchful eyes of their parents. If he had been strong and true, they might be standing watch there, weighing the short-term risks of swing sets against the long-term ones of overprotection, and giving their city-bred kids permission to use outside voices.

As they continue north, they see six-flats marred by chipped mortar and tipped stoops. John used to imagine that the buildings were sinking under the weight of the city's historic crimes. He would make lists of the most egregious, from the extravagant destruction of traditional peoples and pine forests, to the efficient cruelty of hog butchery, to the exploitation of immigrant and African American laborers, to the circulation of boredom-is-excuse-enough violence. He is glad to see that the area looks better than it did when he first came not long after the riots of sixty-eight. He sees quiet courage renewing itself against all odds in the century-old buildings around them, and hopes the flow of history is carrying them away from collective misery.

A few blocks on, John and Melissa emerge from a shady avenue to thread the traffic of 53rd Street at its busiest time of day. They continue north to the building where they lived together during their junior and senior years. Melissa stops and gazes shyly up at the front window of their shared apartment. On his last visit to Hyde Park, John felt nothing when he looked up at that shade-blocked window. Now he feels as if he has come home.

After a pause she says animatedly, "Remember the old gas light fixtures, and the rusty claw foot tub, and the fuses that always blew? I was so impressed that you could fix them!"

John smiles, clasps his hands behind his back, and moves his heels backward onto a patch of turf between the sidewalk and the unbroken line of cars parked at the curb. A harried man in a tight suit rushes by, his sweat coalescing into liquid sideburns.

After a long pause, Melissa asks pointedly, "Don't you remember anything about me?"

"You were a one-woman cottage industry. Our apartment was full of things like those frilly pillows I wasn't supposed to touch!"

"You didn't complain when I made you a down sleeping bag good to minus thirty!"

John's breath quickens. He has hurt her feelings. He has run right into one of his blind spots. His view of life is like a polka dot pattern from the sixties. He replays her lines and sees that he has teased her about a petty irritation when she was looking for lost meaning.

"You were so passionate about movies and books! You made them come alive. And you had a powerful sense of justice. You wanted to set the world right. And when you wanted that, I did too," He adds with a warm smile, which slides into a lowbrow leer, "And I got to live with my girlfriend when a lot of guys weren't getting any."

Her head tips forward. She fixes her eyes on her feet. "I didn't even think of you as a boyfriend. I thought you and I were unique in the world."

His careless lewdness has made her feel cheap. He wants to banish disappointment forever. He wants to remind her of the wholeness of the love they shared, and the beauty of their quest for joy and fulfillment, but the only words he can find are, "I think so now."

They stand side-by-side staring up at the window and into the past. The silence between them becomes a starry sky that contains the answers to all the big questions. Regrettably, John has forgotten how to ask what matters or what's right. Since leaving her, he has sought the approval of those above him in the academic hierarchy, which has meant putting on their values with his white coat and stethoscope, and behaving as if any good comes from the status quo and any harm from bad luck.

Now that he has surged ahead of the herd, though, he has no one to imitate, and must learn to work things out for himself. Some of his near peers have failed spectacularly. An out-of-shape rehab professor tried to climb Everest and fell into a cold hell. Climbers on the northeast ridge route can sometimes spot his body on the ice. The head of Psychiatry lost his job after the fire department extricated him and his mistress-colleague from the wreckage of a Bentley. Their blood alcohol levels were off the charts, but no amount of champagne can explain why they crashed through a Michigan Avenue window displaying their popular feel-good books.

John does not want to turn into tabloid fodder. The good news is if he loses his grip, Melissa will hang on to hers. She doesn't rely on cautionary tales to avoid hubris or self-destructive misery. She doesn't need someone else to set her inner compass toward the good, or to make the moral choices he has lately left to others. And when they are together, they both make better choices.

John is nearly overwhelmed by a powerful upwelling of sweet feeling. He is about to cut it with a tart remark when he stops short. During his medical training, he learned to cut off his wishes and suppress or repress his feelings, which sometimes surface as acquisitiveness or aggression. Just now, he caught a glimpse of his doctor ego reacting to feeling with covertly masochistic self-contempt. It must be on constant alert for threats, which serves him at work but makes it impossible for him to know himself.

John steals a glance at Melissa's face and has a downbeat epiphany. When he is with her, no part of him feels threatened. Even though she turns his world upside down, and persuades him that things he thought right a few hours ago are wrong, he trusts her instincts, which are like those stored in the deepest recesses of his mind. As their minds come into sync, she is helping him in ways he did not foresee. He is thinking in ways he had forgotten, seeing into blind spots, and turning toward the big questions.

"Aristotle said that love is one soul living in two bodies."

"He said the same thing about friendship. Ancient Greek

had several words for love, like philos. Brotherly love. They had a better understanding of the heart than we do."

"Perhaps, but you and I had something more than philos."

John looks up and down the street at the rows of trees on either side, and at the infinite regress of leaves stretching into the distance. At the end of every harsh winter, the irrepressible trees offer new life to the city of dead bricks. Now they remind him that neither life nor love disappears into nothing.

A bus squeals to a stop at the corner. A string of passengers files out. Last to descend is a young man in baggy clothes with a comb sticking out of his hair and a faded old woman on his arm. Melissa stares at them until they disappear down the street.

She takes a raggedy breath and asks, "So what do you do for fun?"

"I should confess right up front that I don't do anything but work. I haven't seen a movie or played the sax in years. And you can see the book I'm reading." He holds out his empty hands, which have stopped sweating now that the day is cooling.

She looks horrified. She tries to joke but can't get the edge out of her voice. "I see. You can feature that in your alumni update: alive but not living."

She gestures southward. With a last wistful look at the apartment, they fall in step and walk to the corner and then turn east on 53rd Street.

They talk of how optimistic a sign it is for the future of Hyde Park that so many shops look up-to-date. Melissa jokes lightly, easily matching John's lifting mood. When they see the new wrought iron balconies and wooden shutters of Beaulieu's New Orleans Bistro, however, she gasps and rushes ahead. She stops at the window and frowns at the elegant linen-clad tables inside.

"Oh, my God! It's beautiful! But it's so wrong!"

"Jerome's changed with the times. I admire that."

Melissa frowns and steps over the threshold into a fictional New Orleans, where they wait in the low-lit, half-full dining room, the atmosphere of which is disturbed by clattering silverware and the scattered energy of a frantic busboy. Melissa stares warily at the upscale clientele and the revealed brick walls and crosses her arms. "When we got here in the 70's, missing plaster meant there'd been a riot, not a remodel. I'll try to like it, for your sake, but it's so commercial!"

"The old Beaulieu's was commercial, too. We grew up with it, so we took it as natural, but it was just the style of the times."

A bored young woman, whose heavy makeup is like a disguise, shows them to seats at a table at the front window. They open the menu books and scan the elegantly scripted list, which is printed on crisp parchment paper. John takes a cold sip from his ice-filled water glass and says, "Guess who the manager is?"

"I give up."

"Jerome Junior."

"No! Didn't he go to the lab school? I thought he'd go on to bigger and better things."

"He's doing what he loves," John says wistfully.

"He's wiser than we are."

"It's never too late."

"Hi!" says a bright voice.

Melissa and John look up. Sarah is standing next to the table, and Doug is standing behind her. "Are you two just in from Monaco?" Melissa asks with a grin.

Sarah and Doug exchange puzzled glances. Sarah looks down at her sun-bronzed skin and the hot pink sun blouse and white shorts that set off her sculpted muscles, perfect posture, and long blonde braid. She laughs and gives theatrical air kisses to Melissa and John. "Doug could be, but I'm fresh from the camper van in my sister's farmyard."

Sarah sits beside Melissa, and Doug stands over the table, a sly grin on his face. He is slender and dressed in stylish black jeans, a rock band t-shirt, and a leather jacket that he slings over his shoulder. From the jacket the eyes of a pair of painted grey wolves seem to follow Melissa. Doug is poised to make a smart remark but a ripple of emotion passes over his face and he picks up Melissa with a bear hug. Then he sits and jokes, "I can't believe we're still eating in this joint."

Sarah and Doug start talking at once and soon chaotic conversation fills the glassed-in storefront with new energy. As they settle in to look at the menu, Melissa asks Sarah, "Are you living in D.C.?"

"Ah. Well. I have a story about that."

Jerome Junior comes to the table and stands beside John who says, "The line sometimes goes all the way down the block! Yours is the hot ticket in town."

"Anytime you want a table, you let me know. We look after our regulars."

"It smells delicious," Melissa says, warming to the surroundings. "Is your Dad here?"

"He's in the back making gumbo. He wants to add fried chicken, but I doubt our customers will go for it. We get a lot of doctors here, thanks to you John, and they don't eat the fried foods."

"What do you recommend for my guests?" John asks.

Jerome speaks to each in turn and then takes the menus and sends a waitress to the table with coffee and hot water for tea.

Melissa says to Sarah, "Tell us the whole story."

"Well, the *whole* story would begin with my graduating with a master's degree in social work and getting a job at the National Center for Health Statistics. I worked my way up, met a guy named Phil who worked in another agency, and we settled down to be a minor power couple. Elections went by, directors changed, and changed, and changed again, and finally one came in who didn't know what she was doing and didn't want to."

John shifts uncomfortably. "Did you speak to her?"

"I tried, but she was very well connected and didn't have to listen."

"What was your salary?" John asks.

"Great, John, but believe it or not, I had taken the job to change the world. Not surprisingly, it changed me. I could protect my division from the new director, but I couldn't protect myself. I lost all faith in management when she imposed one fad after the other—from matrix management to team building to total quality management. She was like those women who change their dresses every few hours. We called her the total appearance manager. Anyway, I knew that she was wasting my time, but I couldn't say how much, so I came in one Saturday morning and measured it."

"How very quantitative of you!" Melissa laughs, her eyelids crinkling.

"How like my work. Anyway, I retrieved every document my division had produced during the preceding two years, from neatly bound reports to sticky notes; divided them into three piles: reports, supporting documents, and wasted efforts—e-mails about failed reorganizations, internal proposals that went nowhere, reports we didn't act on—all of it. Then I used my calendar to tote up the time I wasted in meetings."

"How did you assess that?" John challenges.

"I looked at the minutes and included meetings with no action items. The first cut made it look like the director was disappearing half of my fifty-hour workweek—which would have made her a real magician! But then I took into account the fact that most of our reports were commissioned to make it look like the legislative branch was taking action when it wasn't, which meant that I was wasting forty-nine out of fifty hours a week, for which I was paid for forty."

Doug says to John with a smirk, "Any of your underlings try that?"

"Not that I know of!" John says with an uneasy laugh.

"So," Sarah continues, "I could either stay and keep my chair warm, which is what most long-term employees do, or quit. So I quit, and went up to Lake Cayuga to stay with my sister. I started taking yoga, and soon I was helping the teacher. And I'm hoping to become a partner in her business."

"How wonderful!" Melissa says.

Sarah's face opens in surprise. "I thought you'd tell me off like you used to! That's why I didn't call before."

"She used to have standards," John frowns.

"She still does," Sarah says. "In spite of her illness."

"What illness?" John asks sharply.

"Sarah! I asked you not to mention it!" Melissa exclaims.

"I read those emails. But John should know. He might be able to help."

"You don't understand! Internists hate patients like me!"

"That's ridiculous," John says.

"I have chronic fatigue syndrome."

John feels a surge of disgust. He can feel Doug and Sarah's eyes boring into him, and the painful grip of Missy's shame. There is a thick silence.

"Did you feel that?" Missy asks Sarah.

Sarah nods. "Like a force field."

"What?" John asks irritably.

"Your energy. You've shut her out. And all of us."

John looks at Doug sharply and asks with visible contempt, "Do you believe all this woo-woo stuff?"

Doug replies as if from a great distance. "I live in California. I know my woo-woo. This isn't woo-woo. This is an opportunity for medical research."

"Who would fund it?"

"You would."

John snorts and looks at his friends suspiciously. "Did you plan this ambush?"

Doug looks at Sarah. "Did we plan to ask an old friend that we love to help the love of his life?"

"Didn't have to." Sarah puts her hand on Missy's arm. "Comes naturally."

John sighs and stalls for time. "What have you done so far?" he asks Missy briskly before averting his face toward his empty plate.

"Not much. I can only think clearly when I'm around someone like Sarah, who knows how to refine and share energy. Please don't roll your eyes. I can't talk to you about my reality and protect you from it at the same time."

"Sorry," John says, looking at Doug for support and finding none. "Please go on."

"I started knowing that medicine had already failed me and

that the answers wouldn't be seen or uncovered in the places where people were already looking. So I started on a spiritual journey and developed a series of contemplative practices."

"Like Newton, and other early moderns," says Doug.

Melissa sighs in relief. "Yes! Exactly. Most spiritual practices are about being and becoming, and most religions are about social continuity. But Talmudic and Kabbalistic studies are about God. *They're* about looking into the unknown and seeing and discovering the new. It obviates post-hoc reasoning and avoids forced consensus."

"Isn't it for Torah study?" Sarah asks.

"If you define Torah broadly—say as creation, as Einstein did—you can bring it to bear on anything. I've had some success mixing observation and inquiry through esotericism, but I can only go so far by myself. The process of non-ideological dialogue is for two complementary minds." Melissa's eyes meet John's.

He says, "Like ours were?"

"Like ours. Like soul mates."

"You realize that this has nothing to do with medical science as I know it."

"Yes. It's more philosophical than mechanistic or algorithmic. It blends theology, field biology, psychology, and medicine. It crosses boundaries—all of them."

"Confess," Doug says. "You're curious."

"I'm employed."

"You're going on sabbatical."

"This is just what you need," Sarah says.

John's face contracts.

"What's the matter?" Missy asks in alarm.

He breathes more than speaks. "I've got the world on my

back. I can't do more."

"So quit," Doug says pitilessly. "Why the fuck do you work in medical research if it doesn't burn your jets? Anyone can be a bureaucrat or a manager. For you it's a waste of time. A waste of your life."

John gets up, chair scraping the floor, and walks out. Melissa runs after him. He turns and confronts her. "Why didn't you tell me before? Looks like I need to hold *you* responsible!"

She begins to cry. "I just wanted to be the old me for a day. Just one day. Every other day I'm my illness. It's hell."

John takes her in his arms.

She sobs. "I was holding you responsible for a phone call. My body is holding me responsible for doing the job that our profession is failing to do."

"Our profession *is* failing. Not in responding to trauma or heart disease or cancer or stroke. In being human."

"Yes."

"We have to break free."

"Yes. But after dinner," she jokes, looking into his eyes with the old expression of love.

He feels it now. He sees the light of her soul and feels it trapped inside. He can't say no. He won't. "This is why we did it, isn't it? Went into medicine?"

"Yes."

"And we know how. We learned together."

"Yes."

He follows her inside. Doug and Sarah look at them warily and then relax into eating the food that arrived while Missy and John were outside. The conversation rises again with the usual light gossip about work and family and the serious news about aging parents and alumni and faculty who died too young. All too soon, it seems to Melissa, they have finished and paid and are lingering out front under the streetlights.

"Where are you two staying?" Melissa asks Sarah.

"Doug's been at John's for a couple of weeks, and I'm hoping to stay with you tonight, and then go home with you to Denver and take a yoga teacher training course in Nederland."

"I'd love that!"

"But right now," Sarah says with a keen look at Doug, "I'd like to go out. I haven't been to a city in too long!"

"John?" Doug asks. "Missy? Take in some music?"

"Another time would be great," Melissa says.

"I gotta get back. I've got an early morning," John says with regret.

Melissa gives Sarah her lodging information and she and John watch them walk away into the night teasing each other. Melissa asks, "Are they on again or off again?"

"I think Doug's hoping that they'll be on again after tonight."

"Does his wife know?"

"Apparently. He's always saying that he loves her money and she loves his—"

"—and all his marriage needs is for him to sleep with Sarah—"

"—until they have to take a break."

"How are you and Laurel doing?"

"Bad. The worst it's been. It's spilling over into my work life. That's why Doug's here."

Melissa sighs. "I'm sorry to hear it."

"You and Dan?"

"Bad, but no worse than usual."

John's self-discipline snaps. In his first spontaneous act in twenty years, he lunges at Melissa and holds her as if for the first or last time. He has the dizzying feeling that their spirits are spiraling up through the twilight sky to the stars high above the city lights. He kisses her passionately, oblivious to the hard-shelled South-siders who pass them without a glance. Her body relaxes into his: her mouth, her breasts, her thighs, and, finally, her navel. Past and future disappear. He realizes, with exquisite joy, that maturity has made him more aware of the rich delight of loving a mate who is also a soul mate.

After a time, he pulls away, takes her hands in his, and says ardently, "Marry me! Don't let my stupidity ruin the rest of our lives!"

Shaking her head stiffly, she says with a catch in her voice, "If only you'd asked me twenty years ago, before we both had families!"

"It isn't too late to be true!"

"This is all too precipitous. You don't know what you're doing," Melissa looks into his eyes and says in consternation, "You're completely lost now, aren't you?"

He feels shock that becomes a wave of rage that breaks and collapses when he realizes that her eyes are looking straight into the buried parts of his psyche, the ugly places that even he can't bear to see. And yet she loves him warmly and steadfastly and unsentimentally.

Her voice turns desperate. "Promise you'll play your saxophone this week! If you won't do it for yourself, do it for me. Please!"

He wants her to love him fiercely. He wants love that cuts through pretense and confusion and disarms control. He wants it, but he is not ready for it. "Take it easy."

"The John I knew could handle any truth."

"That kid thought he could do anything. By himself."

"You can do anything. You've forgotten what a wonder you are under all that bluster, and how amazing you are when you aren't blinded by ambition."

"I haven't forgotten what a wonder you are. Don't leave me without hope! I'm offering myself unconditionally. If you won't leave him, think about an affair! We can meet and make love all day or all weekend. It can be our secret."

"You said you'd help me find out what's wrong."

"I will."

"That has to come first. Please. As friends—soul friends. Think about it." She pulls her hands free and backs away. "If you say yes, I'll contact you."

"Yes, of course, yes if—if you'll think about my—what I asked."

Melissa's face contracts into a red knot around piercing eyes. "How will I think of anything else?" She turns and runs, fast, around the corner and out of sight.

2

Caught

For several years now, John has been plagued by the recurring thought that his life—which is like a perpetual whitewater run—has become caught on a snag. No matter what he does, or how efficiently he does it, he can't get clear of the living nightmare in which he is going nowhere. He is burned out. He put off his sabbatical too long. He makes it his New Year's resolution to set up a regular golf game as soon as the snow melts, and to plan a year of study to begin in July. Despite his continuing determination to fulfill his resolution however, he can't seem to do it. Too many urgent tasks delay the important ones. If he does what matters most, he may tip the canoe of his life and drown.

At two o'clock on an April afternoon, the spring before his reunion with Melissa, John leans over the L-shaped desk in his spacious corner office and takes a bite of his daily roast beef sandwich on rye. His eyes avoid the University of Chicago alumni chairs that remind him of his next meeting and the printed papers stacked on tables, cabinets, and bookshelves that remind him of the mushrooming of medical data. *So far, I'm keeping up.*

John chews as he checks his pager, his personal data assistant, the 140 messages in the inbox on his desktop computer, and his pager again. When he has one minute to go, he opens his laptop and logs onto his private account to find Melissa's message waiting in the queue. He has been looking for it every day for a month. It is too long to read now. He flushes, shuts the laptop lid, and throws the rest of his lunch into the trash just as the door opens.

His youngest colleague enters, her face eager. "Dr. Laughlin?"

She looks sixteen. He doesn't bother to ask her to call him John. "Come in. Have a seat." He gestures genially toward a chair.

Over the next several hours, as the chairs empty and fill again and again, John speeds through his workday like a timing belt with digital doodads, finishing on time thanks to his punctilious secretary, Evetia, who guards the outer office as if it were a top-secret military installation. Her angry eyes and long nails intimidate supplicants and protect him from frivolous requests. He waits until she takes home her keen eyes and ears and then opens his laptop to read Melissa's message. She has agreed to come to the U of C reunion in September. He takes a moment to feel the keen pleasure—or is it relief?—of having maneuvered her exactly as he pleased.

On Wednesday morning, John parks his car in its plum spot in the parking garage. He zips into the hospital corridors and onto his research lab, which is buried deep inside the complex close to the MRI machine, the storage freezers, and the other facilities that support cutting edge research. No Chair he knows takes as much time for research, but John couldn't do without it. It gives him the chance to cut through confusion, complexity, and compromise and to glimpse the fundamental order of things. Its golden moments of discovery can propel him through months of wrestling one intractable problem after the next.

John pulls open the door of his lab. A whoosh of unfiltered air passes in. He crosses the threshold into the rarefied suite like a monk entering a sanctuary. The rows of lab benches form a pattern like a giant circuit board that connects an intricately ordered series of apparatuses, humming fans, and workers intent on ritual tasks. He breathes in the air of ascetic devotion and smiles.

John waves lightly to Colin, who manages the thirty investigators, staff, and students who belong to the lab. Colin is standing in a glass-walled room to the left, orienting a new technician to a tabletop electrophoresis apparatus. John nods to a Chinese postdoctoral trainee whose English hasn't improved in three years, raises an eyebrow at a shrouded tissue culture project belonging to a medical student who needs supervision, and suppresses a grimace at the latest lip piercings of a pretty animal technician who is sacrificing her face along with the rats.

John doesn't like the ritual of rat sacrifice, but he accepts it. As he passes the odorous rat room he peers into its recesses. Bloody entrails trigger a memory of the night when he saw hungry South Side children cooking rats over a fire in a metal drum. The suffering of hunger and all the other suffering he has witnessed in the course of medicine form his guidebook to the unknown. He does not wander in that landscape. He does not flip a coin or guess which way to turn. He sets his compass in the direction of basic truths that promise to improve the everyday lot of his species.

He enters his windowless back office. A lone stack of printed sheets sits in the center of his bare metal desk like an offering. He scoops it up with a tingle of excitement. It is the final draft of the new manuscript in which he and Colin report the discovery of a neuropeptide called polycoleptin. Their experiments prove that this peptide can make obese rats lose weight, and imply that it may do so in humans. Colin must have worked on it late into the night.

John slides his briefcase onto the desk and sits down to turn the stark pages with care. Colin has polished it smooth as a cabochon-cut gem. John sits back and savors this moment, which may be the pinnacle of his career.

After publication, John and his competitors will move to develop polycoleptin analogue pills for use in humans, which could help doctors and patients around the world, and produce unprecedented profits for pharmaceutical companies. Publication will also change his life. He will be in a position to bring new research dollars into his lab, his Department, and his University, or, perhaps, to parlay for a choice position in Denver.

"How is it?" asks an anxious voice behind him.

John turns to see Colin's shaved head and Stan Laurel expression hovering above a faded black T-shirt and torn jeans, the uniform of Colin's monastic existence.

"It looks great. We're going to blow them out of the water. But I think we should emphasize the limitations of our assumptions and inter-species generalizations."

Colin blanches.

"Sorry to raise this now. I guess I'm having a philosophical moment."

"You've had a lot of those lately, haven't you?"

John tries vainly to recall what he did to prompt that remark. "Look, I don't want to hold you up. We can always submit it and wait to see what the reviewers say."

"I didn't mean that in a bad way. This paper will make us the leaders in the field. We should set the highest possible standards for ourselves."

John smiles. Colin is no corner-cutting cynic. It is one of the reasons John relies on him. "I'll leave it to your discretion. I have every faith in your integrity and competence."

Colin reddens, mumbles thanks, and rushes out. John hears Colin enter the next office, drag his chair across the floor, and clack away at his computer keys. John can hear Melissa admonishing him for being too stingy with praise. John wonders how things will be for his children, who receive so much of it that he doubts they will be able to endure the self-doubt and uncertainty entailed in a quest for truth.

On Thursday morning, John's watch alarm goes off, signaling that he is due in clinic. He shuts his laptop, checks his belt to be sure he has his pager, phone, and personal data assistant, packs his briefcase, and speeds out of the office to the controlled chaos of clinic. There, he dashes into his exam room and puts on his white coat and stethoscope.

For the next few hours, he thinks of nothing but his patients, who, as chance would have it, are all Gold Coast retirees or downtown employees with stooped posture and large bellies. All have warning signs of high cholesterol, high blood pressure, and high blood sugar. All are sedentary overeaters. All fear cancer, heart disease, and diabetes. None can change the habits that are propelling them toward such ends. Each has failed every treatment John could come up with: diet, exercise, counseling, even hypnosis. They seem to be waiting for his polycoleptin pill.

Later, the only patient John remembers clearly that day is the last, a salesman named Mr. Hernan who is barely able to shift his spherical body onto the examining table. His massive, tailor-made blue and white striped shirt is dark under his breasts, arms, and bottom chin. He pants and pulls out a handkerchief to dry the sweat trickling down his freckled forehead. His lips open between bulging burgundy cheeks. He flashes a cosmetically whitened smile. "Hiya doc!"

John smiles back. He has always liked Mr. Hernan. Everybody does.

Mr. Hernan continues amiably, "You going to fix me up this time?"

Something inside John snaps. He remembers Mr. Hernan's first request, which was to get to the bottom of his inherited "glandular" problem, for which tests were negative. Since then he has failed at even the most minimal of interventions, like putting down his fork between bites.

John drops his usual formality. He puts his hands on Mr. Hernan's shoulders, looks him in the eye and asks, "Do you really think I can lose your weight for you?"

Mr. Hernan's expression clouds up. After a minute, it turns sunny. "Well, somebody's got to help me, don't they, Doc?"

John feels like a traffic signal on the blink. His intentions are in a muddle. By old-fashioned standards of doctoring, John should solve the problem any way he can, even sugar shots, horror stories, or collusion with the family. By late modern standards, he should avoid the old magic of medicine and keep to the center of the herd. To leave it is to risk legal and monetary punishments for him and for the whole hospital.

John loses patience with late modernity. "Are you ready to do whatever it takes?"

Mr. Hernan replies uncertainly, "Sure, Doc. That's why I'm here."

"I'll have the surgeon staple your stomach right now."

John gives Mr. Hernan a brochure. As Mr. Hernan leafs through it, a light of delight comes into his eyes. John realizes too late that he has foregone the old magic for the costly and dangerous fantasy of technological triumphalism, in which the latest procedure will catapult Mr. Hernan out of his life of sloth and gluttony into the starring role of a soap opera full of peril and rescue. John sighs. At least he is doing something that may dissuade Mr. Hernan from overeating.

John calls the surgical resident and has the clinic nurse arrange an emergency stomach stapling. As Mr. Hernan waddles away, John hangs up his clinic coat with regret. He shouldn't violate the carefully orchestrated, fragile procedures that keep the hospital running in all its complexity, especially as it is his job to enforce them. The Chief of Staff will hear about John's spurious emergency, probably from the nurse at the desk, who stares warily at John as he exits.

John senses that he is not himself, but does not know what to do about it. As he waits for the elevator, he tries to look at the clinic through Melissa's eyes. *Missy, are we wise or foolish to take responsibility for those who won't help themselves?* When the elevator opens with a chime, he forgets to wait for a reply.

John speeds smoothly through the rest of his day, holding standing meetings with senior staff and tying up loose ends. As he exits, he loosens his tie and thinks with pleasure of the paper that Colin will fax to Nature tonight. They will hit the ball out of the park with this one. They will take the pennant.

John could even use this coup to move his lab to Denver. He knows for a fact that Colin would give his right eye to live in Boulder. John could even get Colin a professorship there, if he played his cards right. As John jostles through downtown traffic to the expressways, he thinks of Melissa's message.

The lawyer of his mind goes to work on reuniting with Melissa, but before it can speak, a voice in the balcony of his mind calls out an objection. *What about your marriage?* That thought makes John so nervous he nearly sideswipes an old clunker with his fancy foreign sedan. He is driving in two lanes at once. He eases out of one the way he would like to ease out of his commitment to Laurel if he could justify it.

They were satisfied for a few years. Laurel was the trophy wife who advanced his career; he was the meal ticket. He provided money and she provided every other service, including some fairly raunchy sex during which John had to think of Melissa to climax. Everything seemed fine until one Sunday last year, while he was reading the paper, when he saw from Laurel's cold way of serving his coffee that their careful cordiality had degenerated into mutual dislike. His reality split in two. One part went on as usual, and the other began to dream of suing for divorce.

As John enters the Eden's Expressway, he realizes that he doesn't want to go home. The lingering tastes of science and soul love make it difficult to return to the bitter business of deals, machinations, and compromise of which his marriage is a part. This evening, Laurel will cook dinner for the Chairmen of Surgery and Pediatrics, who are coming over with their wives so that the three Chairmen can connive to assault Medical School rules. If they win, they will divert millions of dollars from weaker departments to their own.

John rolls down his car window and lets the cold air distract him from his discontent. He bucks up and backs into the role of player. He switches on the radio to pick up mass media talking points to pepper the conversation. As he approaches his Wilmette driveway, he confirms that the gardening service tidied the yard, and admires the street appeal of his home. Laurel found the cottage while he was still in training. When property values rose, she had a builder turn it into a handsome two-story Cape Cod home copied from a magazine.

When John enters the kitchen from the garage, and tosses his pager into the countertop basket by the door, he watches her talk to the caterer she lured away from a next-door neighbor. On occasions like this, she wears her extravagant emerald jewelry, and people say that her full lips, deep-set eyes and auburn hair are beautiful. Even John can see that her recent eyelid tuck has left her looking good as new.

John questions Laurel closely. She has thought of everything. She has even sent the children to her parents' house for the night. He is amazed at how well she raises them with almost no help from him. Yes, he reflects as he ascends the curving staircase to shower, the first phase of his adult life has been a triumph. His marriage has served it well, and has therefore been a success.

After showering in the marble-lined master bath, John stands naked in front of the slightly steamed mirror and watches his manhood shrivel as cold air moves up his legs. He looks the same as he did on the day he met Melissa, or the day he left her. His jaw is thicker, and the hair on his temples and chest is graying, but he is still the best of the best—and on a grander stage.

A part of him believes this and another part is evident in an expression of panic that jars him back to the present. He struggles to regain control. Tonight he will have to win friends and influence people, wield the power of positive thinking, bend like a reed in the wind. He will have to do his job as Chairman for the sake of all those who depend on him, including the junior faculty and research associates and fellows and residents he has never let down. He can do this. He always summons his confidence.

When he dons the dress clothing Laurel laid out for him on the king-sized sleigh bed, he looks in the mirror again and sees the Chairman of the Department of Medicine, once the youngest in the country, and still rising. He pulls up his bony chest, trots down the stairs to prove he is fit, and goes to the kitchen to help Laurel, who ignores him.

Dinner goes extremely well. Laurel has dressed the simple dining room with yellow roses, and arranged for a trendy meal with fiddleheads and squash blossoms that everyone admires and no one enjoys. She has put on a gauzy dress to comple-ment her hair and jewels. She is the star of the show. The other wives are trophies, too, each in her own way. The wife of the Chairman of Surgery is still the gorgeous blonde bombshell who can make anyone laugh, and the matronly wife of the Chairman of Pediatrics lends her boyish husband the gravitas he lacks. John fulfills his duties as host by sharing stories from the news, edgy ones to set the mood for strategizing.

After dessert and coffee, Laurel dismisses the men to John's cherry-paneled study for whiskey and cigars. He wonders idly if she got that idea from a movie. It can't have been from her father, a beer-drinking coal miner from West Virginia, or John's father, an unpretentious teacher from Steven's Point, Wisconsin. He imagines that the affectation is, like the emeralds she wears, a talisman against her deep-seated fear of poverty.

After John hands out cigars from the humidor, and while he is still pouring glasses of fine Scotch whiskey from the mirrored wall bar, a call takes Jake, the Chairman of Pediatrics, away on an emergency involving a friend's child. He will be gone for at least an hour. He leaves John alone with Leon, the Chairman of Surgery, who is a tall, powerfully built man with veins in his temples and gray hair that forms a stripe around the back of his head. He was an athlete in his youth and is still proud of his bulk. Even at sixty, he shows a compulsion for competition that makes John look lackadaisical.

Leon lounges in one of the espresso-colored leather armchairs that face each other in front of the fireplace, stretches out his long legs, and says, "That Laurel is really something."

John rubs his chin thoughtfully. He has played the game of sexual titillation over wives, but would like to avoid Leon's situational vulgarity, which knows no limits. "Yeah, she sure is."

Leon blows out a puff of smoke and fixes his eyes on John's. "Something on your mind, John?"

Leon is fishing for something. John isn't sure what it is. He tells himself that sometimes the best strategy is no strategy. "I've been thinking I made the wrong choice."

"I didn't think you had the confidence to admit a thing like that. Laurel giving you a bad time in bed?" Leon's lascivious patter is like a polyurethane coating over his raw aggression. It is both tough and transparent.

John slides into the other armchair. "Oh, no. She gives me whatever I want."

The Chairman fondles his cigar with his tongue.

"I got an e-mail from an old girlfriend." John downs his whiskey, which he doesn't like, and sets down his glass. He hopes his grimace is hiding the flush he feels at the thought of Melissa.

"She wants to see you?"

John shakes his head.

"She beautiful?"

John shakes his head. He wonders if Leon's curiosity comes out of boredom or calculation.

"What did you like about her, then?"

John is surprised to find a ready reply. "She was a real spitfire. Just when I thought I had everything figured out, she'd show me something I didn't know, or didn't want to know. She once said to me, 'John, I won't accept anything less than your best.'" John hears Laurel's laugh echo up from the basement through the heating duct. The wives must have moved to the family room. *Why don't I love my wife?*

"What was she like in bed?"

John doesn't want to talk like that of Missy, but the muted barking of a neighbor's Irish setter reminds him of a story that seems harmless. "When she came, the dog next door would howl, or the cats in the alley would screech. Sometimes she'd start laughing and couldn't finish."

Unexpectedly, the lustful Chairman is silent. He frowns and shifts his cigar.

Silence induces John to share a confidence. "She surrendered to me so completely and so passionately. I felt like I was the only man in the world. When she was under me, I flew."

The Chairman pulls out his cigar and asks with a wicked grin, "So what did she see in you?"

John smiles wryly. "I played a lot of music. Sax mostly, and blues harp down at the Hive with Muddy Waters."

The Chairman's eyes light up with something, maybe envy. They talk for a bit about Muddy and his big heart and his funeral, and then Leon continues, "So, this old flame, she saw you play?"

"You know that age. You have nothing but the world is your oyster. We were happy on the town, happy at home, happy in bed."

The Chairman nods soberly. "What ended it?"

"I did." Regret stabs John's heart. He covers it with bluster. "We planned to go west for med school, but I chose to stay, and while she was gone I saw it wouldn't work. Take tonight. Laurel did a great job. Missy would have asked me what I was making for dinner!"

The Chairman chews his cigar and puts on a sober air. "I was in love like that once. It nearly ruined me. I'd stand over the sterile field, scalpel in hand, unable to find the landmarks or make an incision. I'd be thinking, *What is she doing now?*" He glances protectively at his hands. "I wanted her every minute. I could have killed somebody. I nearly did."

Leon wants me to stay with Laurel. Why? John senses a blind spot. He chews his cigar and stares into the cold hearth. Leon's tone is familiar, almost fatherly. John has never seen Leon like this. Perhaps Leon wants to step out of the role of competitor and into the role of mentor. It's time he did. John considers trusting Leon, but old habits of caution hold him back.

"You play golf, Leon?"

Leon does. He invites John to play a round at his club. They talk golf until the Chair of Pediatrics returns, after which they talk strategy until the wives bring out the coats.

"I'm awake," growls ten-year-old Eric.

Melissa ignores the smelly clothes and dusty books on the floor by his bed and focuses on the spidery legs and curly black hair sticking out from under the tangled covers. He is an exact copy of Dan. There is no resemblance or simpatico between her and Eric to evince her role in his birth. Later, as he slouches over the kitchen island eating cold cereal and fruit, his nose buried in a six-hundred-page science fantasy book, she marvels at the mystery behind his aquiline profile, single brow and deep-set brown eyes. She has no idea what he does while he is away or what he thinks of anything. She would like to ask him a personal or substantive question, like what he might want to be when he grows up, but knows he would resent it as much as Dan would.

She settles for asking, "Do you need money for lunch?"

When Melissa awakens seven-year-old Aaron, she sees herself in his sandy hair, blue eyes, and square frame. His resilience and tenacity echo hers, and lend ease to their give and take. When he mounts his bike to pedal to primary school, Melissa warns him to watch for traffic. She avoids a compulsion to tell him to avoid bad company, not wanting to put ideas in his head.

When she rushes to leave for work, she sees a postcard lying on a pile of envelopes under the mail slot in the front door. In the weak light of the leaded glass windows, she makes out the words, "Coming your way after the reunion, Sarah." Melissa stuffs a bagel in her mouth, shifts her sons' soccer bags to the other shoulder, and pulls open the door, scattering mail across the Rya rug and oak floor. She shuts the door quietly so as not to wake Dan, who is still sleeping upstairs.

Melissa already has an uninvited visitor: the twenty-year-old idealist who awakened when she heard from John. That idealist's passion for life is interrupting the mental workflow of the forty-two-year-old Melissa, the multi-tasking manager of her family's late modern lifestyle. The lack of time for thought or happiness sometimes seems to her to be the cause of the many ailments that are slowing her down. She fears that she may lose track of one of the many to-do lists over which she has not been able to gain control. Worse, her callow visitor is diverting energy toward the old losses that are stuck in her brain like a clog in a drain.

Melissa soon reaches her shared office at the hospital, a tiny windowless room with a sterile décor of four desks and framed certificates. She puts on her white coat and pager, smoothes her hair, and tells her younger self that the world is barely systematic, which makes it difficult to create coherence over time. Regrets and wrongs accumulate with experience, shading sense and memory with ambivalence and complexity. Life is therefore bound to leave traces of sadness and disappointment. *It would have been the same with John as it is with Dan. I would be sick and he would punish me for undermining his blind faith in his own ability to keep everything under control.*

Her younger self stands steadfast. *That's just an excuse. You're a sellout. When you compromise to join the system, you become part of the problem.*

Her elder self tries to reason with this sophomoric busybody. *I'm lucky to have work that doesn't compromise my ethics. And that I can do two days a week. Even that little bit is becoming too heavy a burden to bear.*

The sanguine statement about ethics is challenged by her first call. Melissa finds the patient lying flat in bed, her head a specter of crinkled skin topped by feathery wisps of white hair. The old woman's labored breathing is nearly obscured by incessant muttering, which is interrupted every minute or so by a startling and disturbing grimace. A distraught gray-haired woman is slouched over the bed rail. Her disheveled hair and stale breath give evidence of an all-night vigil.

"Doctor," she asks desperately, "can you make Mom stop?"

Melissa sees that the gray-haired woman is distressed by the mother's expressions. "She appears to be in pain. I'll see what I can do. How long have you been up?"

The daughter bites her lip and begins to weep silently.

Melissa says kindly but firmly, "Be sure to take some rest."

Melissa briefly examines the mother, who has a central line sticking through the flesh above the collarbone and a feeding tube impaled in her stomach. Down the hall, the medical record tells her that the patient, whose body is ravaged by breast cancer, begged the staff to be allowed to die but was kept alive at the insistence of the daughter, who was unprepared for death. Wondering idly if the daughter's decision was motivated by ignorance or by unprocessed guilt, fear, or anger, Melissa orders an increase in the patient's pain medication and wishes them both well.

Melissa's younger self scolds, *Failing to accept death when it's due isn't ethical, it's a failure of ethics! The day has barely begun and you've already compromised your ethics!* Her younger self adds, *And, you've done worse! You've ignored every feeling that would alert you to the fact that this system is too simple to be wise and too complex to be wieldy. And you're so corrupt you just go along with it!*

Melissa remembers how in college, she admired the efforts of the young and inexperienced to beat back death; in medical school, after seeing the same scenario time and again, she saw denial of death as a failure of nerve, or the last selfish act by a needy child; now she accepts it as the status quo. *It's not up to me. The system is our way of gaining collective experience with death in modern times. Technology requires us to come together to find a way forward.*

Oh yeah? Who's monitoring dehumanization? Who's

countering the chaos created by top-down thinking? This isn't a factory! You've can't hand over life to this cousin of a punch press!

Who do you think I am? I only work here.

Melissa's shoulders slump a little as she goes to her next patient, a burly, middle-aged diabetic who has been in the hospital for months. After an emergency bowel surgery, his intestines formed a network of abscesses, from which fistulae tunneled their way to the skin to drain pus and blood. No doctor can guess the cause of this apparent infection. Experience tells Melissa that he is unlikely to leave the hospital alive, and that no one will ever know why.

Melissa finds the man sitting up in bed, his belly distended like the laughing Buddha, his face a study in pain. She is grateful to have arrived before the patient's brother, a tattoo-covered former mercenary with a punk hairstyle and a combative attitude. Melissa inquires after the patient's needs and writes an order for more insulin. In a desperate attempt to do more to ease his suffering, she adds an order for a new pillow.

The younger Melissa demands, *Why is the medical record so long when you know so little? Why do you tolerate this failure to avert Death when it comes too soon?*

Okay, smarty pants. Tell me what I'm supposed to do about it.

Fortunately, her younger self grows dull and quiet as Melissa scurries to and fro along the polished floors of the glossy-walled corridors, filling routine requests for stool softeners from nurses she doesn't know for patients she will never see again. Gradually, her shoulders rise, her sorrow subsides, and she regains her poise on the razor's edge between the resistance and rigidity of her younger self, and the expedience and laxity that are seducing her with the aid of age and pessimism.

Melissa hurries home for lunch. The bright, white light of the Denver noon has bleached the red from their Colorado brick house. She spots the garage door open in the back. Shielding her eyes as she strides up the drive, Melissa glimpses Dan's bald spot bobbing up and down inside as if suspended in midair. When she is closer she sees him climbing a stepladder propped against the back wall. She watches his powerful back, which was molded in youth by sailing. He is as lithe and appealing as he was on the day they met.

To get his attention she announces, "Sarah's coming to visit!"

"Oh, great, you're here. Hold this."

If she let him he would turn her into the personal assistant he has expected since he first said "nurse, scalpel, please." As he hands down a four-person tent, he asks, "When?"

Pleased that he listened, but eager to avoid the inevitable cross-examination, she takes the tent and says, "I have twenty minutes. Do you want to do it?"

Dan climbs down promptly, and soon they are catching their breath on the hard mattress in the oak-trimmed bedroom. He turns to the yellow wall, brooding as usual, relinquishing any intimacy to his deeply buried dark side. Melissa has given up trying to approach or understand it, and yet she feels it, and is weighed down by it. She wishes she could block it out or meet it differently, but she can only watch helplessly as it swells her rising pool of sadness.

Melissa grabs a chapati wrap from inside the refrigerator and takes it to the car. She turns on a bossa nova tape to cheer herself up and eats as she drives back to Rose hospital, where she reviews all the standing orders of a Dr. Drew who had to leave for a family funeral. The rest of her afternoon disappears into one routine call after the next until it is time to pick up the boys for their soccer games. Because they attend different schools, and play in different leagues at different fields, she spends most of the next two hours pushing through rush hour traffic.

When they get home Dan is cooking dinner. The boys go into the greenhouse addition off the kitchen, which serves as the family room. Melissa races to her basement desk to switch on the computer and search the online white pages for Sarah's contact information. She finds an astonishing number of listings for Sarah Sewell, and more for S. Sewell. She searches out an old alumni directory with a fairly recent number and sprints back upstairs.

They eat at the kitchen island. Dinner is stressful as usual. Dan's nervous tension increases as the evening shift approaches. Eric sulks for mysterious reasons, and Aaron complains about his homework, which is, she hates to admit, mechanical and overabundant. She picks at her dinner, which is a thick slice of dry ham with soggy French fries and lukewarm frozen corn, and wonders if she should replace the stools on which they are sitting, which are so uncomfortable that they add to everyone's edge.

The stools are too expensive and too new to replace.

Stuck again, aren't you? Can't you take control of anything in your life? Have you no shame?

Yes, I have plenty of that. Find something constructive to do.

Melissa is fed up with her younger self, who notices every hidden pothole, cliff, and iceberg, as well as every dust bunny, wooly bugger, zit, and chip. That self is a cross between an angry protester and a white-gloved mother-in-law who is looking to justify her disapproval by finding dust. This chimera is hunting down and collecting all the displeasures retained by her mind. Those on which she dwelt are enclosed in cages and those she ignored turned to swamp creatures in the dark wetland of her subconscious. Each and every one has a life and voice she must comprehend if she is to evolve her losses of love, health, and hope into a new beginning.

She sighs and watches Dan scowl as he finishes his dinner. He is unhappy, too. She has been waiting for years for his permission or participation in their shared happiness, but he never stops reacting to discontent by trying to control more and more and more, which only empowers the exigencies that dictate their every move. If she continues to wait for him, she will be waiting forever. She will have to act on her own. She will have to live a parallel life, at least for a while.

Minutes later, as Dan bustles to the back door, he pulls her aside. "You didn't say much tonight."

"Me!" she exclaims. *Since when do you want me to fill in the blanks?*

Dan chews his lip. "You need to get out. Do something."

"I'd rather do less."

Dan shakes his head and sets his features in a look of disapproval.

"What? What's the matter?"

"It took you years to get over it. Why bring it all up again now?"

Melissa flushes with shame. "I didn't get over anything. It's time I faced it all. And I can face it with the help of my old friends. John's not bad, you know, just overly ambitious."

"I'm not worried about that megalomaniac. I just want to let sleeping dogs lie," Dan growls, crossing his arms. "It affects us all when you get emotional."

She replies decidedly. "It affects me when we pretend everything's fine. It affects me when you take me for granted until you remember to castigate me."

Dan chews his lower lip. "Damn that Sarah. I hope she never shows." He turns away, picks up his black bag, and stomps out the door to work. Dan inevitably brings up difficult topics when he is leaving and can avoid her reply, which is, *Maybe you should deal with your stuff instead of projecting it onto me and trying to keep me from dealing with yours as well as mine.*

Melissa goes back to the kitchen to clean up. As the boys continue their homework, punctuating it with roughhousing, Melissa's elder self justifies the risk she is taking. *I am grateful for what we have, but I mustn't go against myself, especially when it enables our shared weaknesses.*

After the struggles of the day, she resolves to move Sarah's visit to the top of her priority list. When the boys finish their homework, and play a video game, and go up to bed, Melissa goes to the basement to call Sarah. After ten or twelve rings, she hears a man's voice. "Hello."

"Sorry to bother you so late. May I please speak to Sarah?"

"No-o-o." His voice is hoarse with drink or sleep.

"Is this the right number? I got a postcard from her and wanted to get in touch."

"Good luck," he snorts. "She's gone. Moved out."

Melissa is shocked. "She's on vacation?"

"Yeah, a permanent one. I'm having to sell the condo at a loss." He sounds more bothered by the forced sale than by Sarah's absence. Melissa is fairly sure he is drunk. "Are you all right?"

"No, fuck you very much." She hears a click and a dial tone.

Melissa finishes a load of laundry, puts away the dishes, and goes up to bed. She checks on the boys, showers, and lies down to sleep. She can't. She can feel John's love, the way it permeated her soul and strengthened the weak places. She remembers the delicious feeling of filling him as he filled her.

When she first met Dan, she tried to recreate that sweetness by showering Dan with love, but he clammed up, and settled ever deeper into a posture of cold anger that she met with pleasing and pleading.

I am going to have to dig deep and change. Dan will have to deal with it as best he can.

3

Control

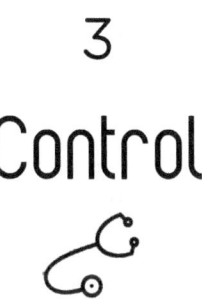

Doug's role in business has evolved with the age of information technology: from start-up partner to acquirer of startups to venture capitalist in search of businesses that will jump-start the new, sustainable economy. He likes B-to-B websites—business to business—especially distribution systems. He views himself as the conductor of a symphony of many parts, each of which he is obliged to improvise as he goes so as to stay at the cutting edge of change. Right now he is enjoying an intermission during which he will critique the old ideas and look forward to trying the new. His gut tells him that this is a good moment, but he has no idea why.

Doug looks around at the flat fields that extend beyond the horizon of thick haze encircling them. He peruses the produce stands crammed on one side of the commuter parking lot, where noisy families are picking over cartons of bright strawberries, pyramids of orange squash, mounds of oranges, buckets full of bouquets, and knobby bags of nuts. The cast of characters crammed into the other half of the lot includes local hangers-on, farm workers, face painters, rug rats, transients, and tourists. It reminds Doug of Cinco de Mayo in the Mission, and of the joys of childfree life.

Doug's latest visionary, Mr. Velasquez, drove him here, way

the heck south of Palo Alto, to pitch Doug in the middle of this fruit and vegetable circus back of beyond. The man must be cracked if he believes the narrow winding road he drove to be the way to the future. If Doug weren't nauseated from the ride, and didn't need a break before the drive back, his irritation would get the better of him and he'd pull the plug on this pitch right now.

"Old people want to eat vegetables now. The men have heart disease and their women want to cook low-fat, low-salt meals. But the supermarket food has no flavor, and it's full of poisons. Remember Alar? That yield-increasing chemical that was used on apples and that was banned because activist moms noticed it was hurting their children? That frightened young mothers. They don't want to ban poisons one at a time, they want to dismiss all of them at once. They want this!" Velasquez says. He sweeps his arm toward the stand behind them, where a pair of young men stares at them surreptitiously between sales.

The young men are not the only ones to notice the tall, black-haired South American who took Doug on this unexpected tour. Velasquez is an eye magnet. He is voluble, earthy, open hearted, and scientific, and he is only getting started. "They don't want to strap their little ones into the car to drive them all the way out here. But look! Think of the trouble they had to take!"

Doug looks at the squawking children streaking around in the lot, running off the lengthy ride. He'd like to do the same. "I'll buy that."

Velasquez takes Doug's elbow and pulls him to a distant stand of dirty fruits and gnarly roots. The South American says something in Spanish to a short, dark, sales woman, picks up a shaggy parsnip that leaves a trail of brown dirt, and lectures Doug about the chemistry and bacteriology of organic soils.

Doug tunes out to take time to size up this oddball. Mr. Velasquez is charismatic. If he weren't, Doug would already be in the car. On the other hand, Doug can't picture the roots of this puzzling pitch artist who wants to come north of the border to reinvent the grocery business. Doug can't imagine the sources of this visionary's passion, privilege, or erudition. Doug decides to reread Borges, Marquez, and Neruda before signing anything.

Doug suppresses his unreasonable irritation. He is irked to be out in the sticks. The only ploy less appealing to him would be an office pitch by a con artist, or by a business school student with a penchant for pie charts. When a visionary calls, Doug always says two things: "I never take a pitch over the phone or in the office," and "If you can't entertain me you'll never get my venture capital—my VC is for people who have fun pursuing their passion."

That policy has its perks. Even the most creative visionaries will stake out a claim to normalcy by taking him to sporting events. Fishing pitches are his favorite because he loves to be out on the water in a boat. Even a dinghy will do. Opera pitches are his least favorite. They are almost always bombastic and usually require him to sit through hours of schmaltz.

"The money all goes into distribution. This is true for cars, movies, energy, food, soap, everything. All of those distribution systems are about to change. They all depend on free oil and the oil is going to run out. In twenty years, people will buy everything on the Internet."

"I'm with you there, pal. It's all about distribution. But how are you going to change that?"

Mr. Velasquez' mouth opens in a laugh. His eyes pierce Doug's. This is a question the man has been waiting for. "Stay-at-Home

Grocer will have a fleet of propane trucks that will go to every house in America! We will be like cable television. We will be first, and we will feed everyone."

Doug has a weakness for this type of vision. He has a Chicago-born belief that wealth comes to cities, not individuals, and that its purpose is to raise the quality of life for everyone. Montgomery Ward, the motive power behind Chicago's public waterfront, is one of Doug's heroes. He has no time for people who worship the past or stuff mattresses with money. He likes the big picture, dynamism, and ideas with the power to shape the future. In his view, we are all in the same boat, which is rapidly expanding to include the entire planet, and is trying its darnedest to sink.

Doug says skeptically, "Reinventing the food market would be a big coup. If you can do it."

He feels the pull of this plan. He likes the idea of serving basic needs, of selling things that always matter, like mortuaries, medicine, and food. The rest is luxury. He likes that food can go both ways. He loves being pitched in Napa or Sonoma, and has been thinking of putting money into a destination vineyard, or a hobby winery of his own.

But he has never considered being a grocer, or promoting a grocer, or even talking to one. "Why here, why now? Why are people ready to make this change?"

Velasquez can barely contain his excitement. He is as pleased with Doug's questions as Doug is with his answers. They are coming to a meeting of the minds, the kind that revs both their motors. "America is the only country that is ready. The people want healthy, farm fresh food. The organic farms are well established. When we have capital, we can expand south."

Doug has inadvertently researched this topic through his

wife, who is a gourmet macrobiotic health freak. She is not a typical consumer, whatever that is, but she shares the general fear of disease. They don't sleep together, but always eat together, even though her excellent cooking comes with a generous helping of repetitive conversation about the reasons organic food should be at the center of everyone's plate.

"What about community supported agriculture, farmer's markets, and co-ops? Aren't they sucking up the supply chains?"

"The supply is expanding rapidly."

Mr. Velasquez has an answer for everything. He has thought it all through. Doug likes that. In his experience, success comes to charismatic visionaries with absolute conviction, and profits go to those with energy, tenacity, perspective, and follow through. Doug thinks this man may be one of those rare alchemists with the potential to turn charisma into an economic engine.

Doug has, in his analytical way, zeroed in on his personal predictors of success. He has never told anyone what they are. They are his bag of magic tricks. If he retires he may write a book, but probably not. He is not a man who likes to put his cards on the table.

One sign is personal grooming. He doesn't care what people wear, but if they smell or look dirty, he doubts their work ethic. This sign works in Protestants, Jews, and even fresh-off-the-boat Asian immigrants who have no faith in anything he knows of. He will, on rare occasions, go for a geek in a garage, but all of the slovenly geniuses seem to have been discovered. Another sign is what some call gut feeling but Doug recognizes as love. He loves certain visions the way other men love some women, or children, or dogs. This feeling tells him he is ready to bet on the vision and to take care of it.

Doug is not feeling the love, at least not as yet. Something about this pitch is bothering him. He takes his time browsing through the bumpy turnips and bruised tomatoes, plastic bag in hand, waiting for this vague bother to speak to him. If it doesn't, he will walk.

Suddenly, as he is staring at an apple, a more urgent memory captures his attention. He is a boy again. His parents are driving him into the countryside on a Sunday in the fall. They are happy. Their hearts belong to the farmland that is still only an hour's drive from their suburban bungalow. That day, they are driving all the way around the south shore of the Lake to Michigan. Finally, they reach the roadside stand of a favorite orchard that sells sky apples and strawberry apples and other fruits he has never seen before.

Doug remembers taking home a tiny, pink sky apple. He is sitting in the back seat of the car. His little brother must be a baby because Doug has the seat and the treat all to himself. When he bites into its crisp, tart, plum-scented flesh, he experiences an epiphany. It melts in his mouth. Its sweetness is only a part of the complex delight of its flavor. He takes tinier and tinier bites so that it will last and last. He can feel it in his hand now. The flesh of the apple isn't turning brown even though he is taking time to suck the juice slowly from each tiny nibble.

"I'm all about distribution systems," Doug says absently.

Doug has the feeling now. He is helpless in its grip. He is only going through the motions. What's more, he intends to gamble his own money on this project so as to have the chance to revisit his earth-covered roots. He can't wait to put on an old flannel shirt, dig his boots into the dirt, pick up a pitchfork, and take a poke at a patch of sod.

He is way ahead of Velasquez now. The only problem is that he can't think of a way to free up a spare bit of capital. All his assets are tied up until the summer. His wife has a money market fund that isn't doing well, but she is much too attached to her local organic grocer to consider investing in this new venture. That needn't be a barrier. What she doesn't know won't hurt her.

The ride back is not so bad. The country is beautiful, and Doug likes Hector Velasquez, who is telling Doug about his other kaleidoscopic visions. Doug's mind begins to wander. He scans the horizon and thinks of ways to get Sarah to wander willingly back into his net. He offered to fly her out and she said yes, but then she changed her mind. He could fly there but that would undermine his image.

Doug has the sense that Sarah wants to say no for good. He will make his move first. Hector's visions inspire Doug to have one of his own. He will use the profits from Hector's venture to buy a condo in wine country that will appeal to Sarah's sense of romance. He will invite her to live in it and set her up with a yoga studio. Doug smiles. Everything is falling into place. When they return to Palo Alto, he'll give Hector a big fat check.

Sarah rises before dawn, as she has done every day since leaving D.C. She bundles up, gathers a stack of blankets, and crosses the gravelly backyard to the scrub-lined creek leading down to Lake Cayuga. The beam of her flashlight breaks over snow-covered rocks and lumps of clay on the frozen path. At the water's edge, she walks out onto the dock; the planks creak; her footsteps echo across the narrow lake. At the dock's end she wraps herself in blankets and sits on a low bench in the fishing shelter built by her brother-in-law's grandfather.

Sarah's opening prayers acknowledge the land, the indigenous peoples who understood it, the Transcendentalists who loved it, and the Quakers who tended it. She gives thanks for Thoreau's study of Hindu scriptures and Emerson's sermons on nature. She visualizes roots extending from her feet into the water, the land, and the near past. The brisk breeze that swirls over the lake's surface reddens her cheeks, but she is warm in her swaddle of down and wool. Sarah soon enters a transparent meditative calm in which she is distantly aware of dawn breaking gradually as gray, flat light behind a cover of low clouds.

When Sarah's watch alarm sounds, she walks up the creek and past the dark red dairy barn and gradually returns to the place between worldly and other worldly awareness that she inhabits in the well-sealed obloid trailer behind the farmhouse, which has become her hermitage. She stops inside to leave the blankets on her bed and then continues around the brick farmhouse to the circular gravel drive in front, where she gets into her sister Maryanne's car to drive into Ithaca for the early morning yoga class. As she drives south on a winding two-lane highway, she sends a blessing to every thing or being that her eye sees. She blesses an elaborately branching oak, a tuft of brown grass piercing the snow, a chevron of birds in flight, a boulder cracked by ice.

As Sarah approaches Ithaca, she feels as if she has been driving through a picture postcard. The rolling hills and barns remind her of the time when horses and buggies went this way. The icy surround, which is glistening now that the yellow sun ball is burning through the thinning clouds, dazzles her eyes. She came to this picturesque countryside for vacation, but here, where she is practicing yoga and helping to care for her niece and nephew, she is on a wondrous, permanent vacation in which she does only those things that increase love and vitality. She is living in a haven that is, for now, a kind of heaven.

At Ithaca, Sarah passes the bus station and the compact old city center, with its new pedestrian mall, and stops near the towering trees of the lakefront park by the small house where her favorite teacher keeps a studio. Crossing its threshold is like entering summer. The students sit on their mats like sunbathers in the simple studio, which is illuminated by golden light and enlivened by multicolored curtains and blue and burgundy yoga mats. Sarah slips off her shoes, hangs her coat on a peg, and goes to the front to greet her teacher. "Namaste."

"Namaste." The owner and instructor, Patricia, who looks larger and younger than she is, pushes her unruly Jew-fro up away from her beaming smile. "Well? Have you decided?"

"Would it be all right with you if I wait until after the next teacher training session?"

"Absolutely. I don't want you to say yes until you're wild with joy to join me. Would you like to assist today? Whatever you decide, experience will help you on your way."

"Yes, thanks."

"Why don't you start by finding out who may need to modify an asana?"

"Be glad to."

Sarah pauses to take a drink from the water cooler. She is tempted to accept Patricia's offer to be partner and successor, but promised Doug to consider his offer of a studio in Napa. Sarah suspects he will lose interest, but is not sure, and wants to wait so as to move ahead without regret. Sarah goes from mat to mat and learns that Judith, a round-shouldered, droopy-eyed therapist of sixty, has rheumatoid arthritis and limited motion in her wrists and ankles. Angela, a dimpled blonde masseuse, has a bad back; Craig, a tall, dome-headed loner, is unable to bend his left knee; and Layla, a wasted woman who appears to have cancer, is fatigued.

This Saturday class is Patricia's gentlest, and therefore the most difficult to teach well. Sarah likes it because she can detect the subtle energies of each pose, and so detect the optimal posture and effort. It is also teaching her how to perceive the unity beyond uniformity, and so to guide each student to find the right angles and effort. She is learning to read body types, personalities, and limitations so as to guide students away from physical and emotional error. Patricia is the ideal teacher to nurture Sarah's ability to give and receive guidance. Patricia is open, perceptive, skillful, generous, and forthright. She is free, and uses freedom well. Sarah's previous instructors, though luminous, were bound by obedience that restricts intuition and instills dependence.

Later, when Sarah is engrossed in arranging a small forest of raised arms and legs, it happens. Her center becomes an empty axis through which energy flows from the collective consciousness above, through her root chakra, and into the earth below. The world of ten thousand cares that revolves around the axis of her spine disappears into a blur. She does not need to be anywhere else or to do anything else. She is at home in her body. Surety radiates from her center. Dissatisfaction is powerless to obscure her perfect equilibrium.

For the rest of the lesson, Sarah remains at the still center of the turning world. When class ends and the others have gone, and she is standing at the door with Patricia, Sarah puts her hand on Patricia's arm and says, "Yes! The answer is yes, yes, yes. You are my teacher. You are the master who can make me a master. I won't waste this precious opportunity that you've offered. I'm ready now to appreciate it, to embrace it, to love it."

Patricia gives her a hug of delight, after which Sarah leaves with a new sense of purpose. She feels exactly as she did when she decided to go away to college at the University of Chicago, and again when she met the wonderful young peers who became her lifelong friends. She made a mistake after that. She chose the wrong path. But the mistake was not in being a strong-willed idealist, or in becoming a part of the massive social machine that many confuse with her country. It was ceasing to learn and to evolve. Her mistake was stasis.

When Sarah reaches the outskirts of town, she whispers, "If it becomes a mistake, I'll change."

On the drive home, Sarah thinks through the logistics of realizing her choice. They are few. Maryanne has already invited her to stay as long as she likes, and to eat with them as often as she likes, which will make it possible for her to live well on a small salary. Sarah parks in front of the farmhouse, glad that it is Saturday so that the children and Maryanne will be home, and Sarah can announce her choice to the family she loves.

She is as happy for Maryanne and her family as she is for herself. Maryanne and her husband, Grant, have taken on far too many responsibilities. Grant works full time as a Dean at Wells College, and Maryanne, though she has a part time job in the Development Office at Cornell, is trying to maintain ideals of family life that evolved when families were far larger, and many hands made light work. She bakes bread, knits, gardens, and takes care of the children, and has radiated happiness since

Sarah came to pick up the slack.

Sarah finds Maryanne in the large kitchen at the back kneading dough for potato bread. The sun is streaming in the window, illuminating her floral dress and long, frizzy, light brown hair, which is gathered in a barrette on her crown. Her little sister's delicate features and curly hair always remind Sarah of Botticelli's Venus, though Venus is fixed, and Maryanne is always in motion.

"Hiya. Want some help?"

"Oh, hiya. Sure! Why don't you see if the kids want to paint now?"

After putting out paints and papers on the kitchen table for nine-year-old Margie and seven-year-old Sam, and collecting them from the living room, Sarah announces, "I have news, everyone. I've decided that after the next teacher training session, I'm going to come back and work for Patricia!"

"Does that mean you'll live in the trailer?" Margie asks.

"Of course she will!" Maryanne says happily.

"Yes. I love the trailer. It's just right for one."

"And it's free," Maryanne adds.

"I wouldn't say that," Sarah replies with a sly smile. "But the price is one I *want* to pay."

Sarah is happy to be able to help. Even though they inherited the farm debt-free from thrifty Quaker ancestors, and lease its dairy barn and east fields to neighboring farmers, and hold down good jobs, Maryanne and Grant barely keep up with expenses. Sarah will not augment their income, but will make their lives easier, and hold down their costs. She and Maryanne have already planned to paint and refurbish the farmhouse, which was built by Grant's great-great-grandfather and is ready for an infusion of energy and ideas.

Later, over lunch, when Sarah tells Grant of her plans, he says, "Stay as long as you like."

She is sure then that she will save him time or money, or both. Grant is unsentimental and ungenerous, except with regard to his children, and would not welcome her unless he felt the balance of time and money tilting his way. "Thanks. The trailer's starting to feel like home. And I love being Aunt Sarah. How did I ever get along without Margie and Sam?"

Sarah loves spending quality time with children she loves, and then leaving them in good hands while she enjoys the perfect freedom of solitude. Later that night, when she has read to the children and kissed them good night, Sarah dashes ten yards to the trailer, which is sitting on cement blocks, and climbs in to sit at the Formica table and write an entry in her journal. A gust howls up the west pasture from Lake Cayuga and rattles the walls and table. Sarah enjoys the wave of wind, which she takes as a sign of nature's exuberance, and rides it by bouncing gently in her seat. She writes:

Basking in being valued. Feeling light and free and full of vitality. Loving the wind and the snow and the lake and the land.

Several pages later, when she has elaborated on the delights of choosing her next path, she looks over the dog-eared volumes propped between two jars of canned dill pickles and marvels at the complicated struggle they detail. When she reads them she is discomfited by the catty teen and conniving adult preserved in their pages. Sometimes, though, she finds them hilarious, and lately, she feels rare moments of conscious indifference that lead her to believe that she may soon be mature enough to leave her journals behind.

Sarah scoops up the journals strewn across the table like a babe in arms and estimates that they make ten pounds. She has written an entry almost every day since seventh grade, when she wrote in a teen diary with flower power decals and a tiny metal lock. The rest of her journals come in all shapes and sizes and colors. They fill half the table, all of the shelf space, and part of a disused bedroom in the farmhouse, but they never helped her to solve the recurring problem of Doug, which must account for thirty pounds of entries at the least.

Sarah used to think she journaled to resolve things, but now she can see that most of the time she was only justifying and rationalizing dubious behaviors. Sarah puts a foot on the cold floor and pivots to the bed, where she settles on a tapestry-covered pillow to meditate on this error. Later, as she falls asleep, she resolves that she will draw the chapter of Doug to a close, end the habit of gossip, and finish every unfinished moment and resolve every unresolved feeling. To enter the eternal now, she must walk the path of purification, which will be daunting, but will lead to an abode of equanimity from which she will be able to look back without obsession, partiality, or regret.

John becomes aware of just how tightly wound his life has been when he begind to lose control of it.

While driving home from work, he is burning to talk with Laurel about taking a sabbatical. He wants to recapture the sense of adventure that he felt when they first set out to homestead in the wilderness of adult life. When he reaches the driveway, though, he is unpleasantly surprised to see a strange car, and then to enter the house and discover Laurel in the middle of an impromptu infomercial for her latest gadget. A family he can't quite recall is watching politely while she demonstrates the floral pattern her new grill makes on both sides of a pork cutlet. When John has hung his jacket in the mudroom, and put his pager in the countertop basket, she says, "Isn't it great that Brett and Celia are here with Tony and Allie!"

Tiffany, a redhead with Laurel's freckles and broad cheek-bones, jumps in front of John, bounces on her tiptoes and announces that she made three base hits in her softball game. Before her father can say a word, she reports that her thirteen-year-old brother Alex was sent home from a friend's house for breaking a lamp. When short, wild-haired Alex rushes in preceded by excuses, she raises her voice and tattles that fifteen-year-old John Junior is playing a forbidden video game in the basement with Tony. Again.

John praises his daughter for her base hits and asks Alex to call Junior. He greets Brett and Celia with polite handshakes and then sends Junior to his room and makes sure that Alex has made amends for the breakage. While Tiffany is still talking, Laurel tells them all to take seats around the dining table. When Alex has fetched Junior, and they are seated, Celia says grace and the children tuck in to finish quickly and be excused to go to the basement family room.

Celia, an angular woman with wary, deep-set eyes turns to Laurel to complain about the prices of her most recent purchases. John steels himself and turns to Brett, an accountant who appears to be made of zeroes. He has oval eyes, round glasses, a dimpled chin, oval cheeks and an oval belly. John comments on the weather, the traffic, the food, and the holiday season. None of these topics engages Brett. Finally John says, "How about those Bears?"

Brett brightens and talks a blue streak about last season's games. John's mind wanders. The table looks great but feels ghastly. He can't imagine what they were thinking when they planned this empty busy life. He wants to leave the table, but wills himself to stay until Laurel and Celia go to the kitchen, and he and Brett are free to go to the basement with the kids and make a power play for the television remote. Brett finds a replay of a Bears game and the children disappear up the stairs.

John wishes he could speed up the clock. When Laurel and Celia come downstairs, he announces that it is time for him to get some shut-eye. An hour later, when Tiffany and Alex are asleep, and John Junior is shut up in his room, Laurel is still peeved. She goes into the master bedroom and then into the stone-lined shower of the master bath. He brushes his teeth, washes his face, and undresses.

When she finally emerges, he watches her smooth a floral scented lotion over her breasts and hips. His middle member thickens. He still finds her attractive. When she walks to the high bed and slips on a satin chemise and boxer shorts, he imagines having sex with her in a far-away place while the children are at school. He goes over, kisses her neck below her ear, and whispers, "How'd you like to spend a year in Rome, or Lyon, or Auckland?"

She grabs a fashion magazine from the cherry side table and crawls under the duvet.

"Laurel, we need to talk," he says firmly.

"You can talk in the morning. It's been a long day."

"I'm going to take that sabbatical in a few months. It'll give us the chance to go abroad, get to know each other again. Think about where you'd like to take the kids."

"Tiffany and Alex have band and Junior won't want to leave his friends."

"Laurel, this is the opportunity of a lifetime. Our children may never have a chance like this again. We've talked for years about how it's one of the few real perks of an academic job."

"I'm not going to leave my life just because you feel like taking a trip."

"Laurel, it's not a trip. I'm completely out of gas."

"Well, mister, you'd better find a way to fill yourself up. You've got me and three kids to take care of." Laurel fights briefly with a tangled sheet and lies down on her side.

John goes into the stone-lined shower stall, turns on the massaging showerhead and stands under its powerful, hot spray. As steam envelops him, his chest tightens and the stall shrinks. Suppressing his rising desperation, John turns off the water, opens the glass door, and stumbles onto the slick floor, where he grabs the towel rack to keep from falling. Panting, he grabs a plush robe and slips it on. He barges through the bedroom and down the stairs to the basement, where he paces wildly.

As Leon pointed out, John is a lucky son of a bitch. But he can't do it any more. He just can't. His life is a prison. It's turning into solitary confinement. He thinks of Melissa and feels a rush of hope. He darts for the stairs and, taking them two at a time, runs up to his study, grabs the phone and sits on the floor cross-legged. He dials the number and holds his breath.

"Hello?"

"Doug?" John asks, his voice tense.

"John?" Doug asks incredulously.

John's chest relaxes slightly. "God, it's good to hear your

voice." John starts rocking and takes a deep breath. "Is this a good time?"

"It's fine. What's up?"

"I need your advice."

"About?"

"My, uh, domestic situation."

"You're asking *me*?"

"It's about my sabbatical. I'm thinking of going alone. I can't stand it here."

"You just answered your own question."

"Right."

"You okay?"

"Good, now. You?"

"Good. Glad to be of help. Call any time."

"Thanks. I will. I … I'm in free fall."

"Don't land before the reunion."

John and Doug talk for a while during which time John relaxes and regains control.

When he hangs up, John stands, puts the phone in its cradle, and creeps down to the basement. He lies on the sofa. That was close. Too close. His expectations are spinning. He has to land somewhere. And soon.

Melissa feels as if the incipient crack in her marriage has yawned open like a crevasse in the spring sun. Now that she has quit work and is looking for a way to do the medical detective work to crack her own case, she sees the marriage as if from a distance—as an aspect of daily life that she must manage before she is free to care for herself.

The marriage counselor holds a folder in her lap and a pen in one hand. She peers at Melissa over pointy half glasses and asks neutrally, "And how does he express his love?"

Melissa looks at the counselor and then looks out of the high dust-edged window at the sun disc trying to get through the gauzy sheet of high clouds. She looks at the African violet on the desk and sees it struggling and feels a pang for it. Then she realizes that she has been looking at the dead leaves and ignoring the living ones. She is being a pessimist. That is a problem she is working on and would like to talk about. "I've been trying to remember the good things, trying to be optimistic."

"Mmm. And how does Dan express his love?"

Melissa thinks of her partner-competitor Dan, who is waiting his turn in the lobby. He didn't tell her he scheduled this dual appointment until he was turning into the parking lot on the way home from the grocery store. As they came in he mumbled something to the effect that she needed to talk to someone. She didn't bother to point out that she has been trying to talk to him for two decades. "You didn't ask if he had any love to express."

The marriage counselor nods. "Go on."

Melissa sighs. She turns in the low easy chair to look around the room. Everything is neutral and natural, including the collage-like leaf prints on the walls, the scattered votives, and the altar of stones and feathers propped against a sidewall. Melissa knows the décor is designed to be calming but finds its blandness depressing, especially in the low light that decolorizes it, as if to enhance night vision that penetrates shadows but makes the world gray.

"Well, he paints the house, and takes care of the boys. He's a very good Dad, very involved."

The counselor leans forward attentively, "Paints the house?"

Is this reflective listening? How silly! "The magic words 'I love you' have never passed his lips. He's a provider. I'd say we're good friends who decided to marry and make a family."

"Mmm-hmm. How would you describe your intimacy?"

"Well, the sex is fine, if that's what you mean. Anyone can have great sex if they want to, can't they? Birds and bees and all."

The counselor recovers her detached voice. "No problems with sexual intimacy, then?"

Melissa pulls a tube of lip-gloss from her purse and applies it. She can see that this woman could benefit from a better knowledge of the mechanics of human sexuality. Melissa fights to stay in the role of patient. "I could come up with one if it's important to you."

The counselor's expression is a blank, but the edges of her nose turn red and her voice grows thin as she says, "How would you describe your emotional intimacy?"

"Well, aside from tension and irritation Dan doesn't show a lot of emotion. Sometimes I think it's there, underneath, but I never know if I'm imagining it."

"And *your* emotions?"

"I've been sad a lot, which is hard on Dan. So, we've been pretty distant lately."

The counselor smiles wryly. "And how would you describe your feelings for Dan?"

"Oohph." That question makes Melissa feel like a husk. "Now you've cut to the chase." She wishes she could see blood on the walls and hear screams from another room. She is frustrated that the body displays its woes so openly, and the psyche so covertly. At the same time, she is loathe to entrust her own shadows to a masked stranger who may have little experience and less depth. "Well, I like Dan. I do. But I'm in love with someone else, an old boyfriend who got back in touch last month. I don't have to guess what he feels. We're soul mates."

"I see. And how does Dan feel about that?"

"He hasn't said."

"Does he know?"

"He must be concerned or he wouldn't have sprung this on me."

"Sprung this on you?"

"He didn't tell me about the appointment until we got here."

"Ahh. Hmmm. And what do you make of that?"

"What do you make of it? I would guess that after years of using me as his Jungian shadow he's decided to get you to talk to me for him."

"What do you suppose he would want me to say?"

"I have no idea. We don't talk, about anything, especially not the tough stuff. Maybe he doesn't want me to leave. Or maybe he does."

"Have you thought of leaving him?"

"Yes, and no. I want things to work out but I want to put myself first now and then, deal with my own shadows and the illness I have that he neglects and the feelings he abuses."

"Shadows?"

"I lost my soul mate, my career, my income, and my colleagues, and most of my friends. Everything but my family. So of course I don't want to lose that. But sometimes Dan makes it intolerable. Quite frankly I think suicide is my best rational option. But I'm passionate about life, so I put myself on antidepressants."

"How does Dan feel about that?"

"I wish that he would face that question and work his way through it. I don't want to be his mother or his recalcitrant patient. I want to be his wife, and he doesn't seem to know how to husband me. Or doesn't want to."

"I see." The counselor's face relaxes into a long, slack-jawed oval. "Is there anything else you'd like me to know before I speak with Dan?"

"Well, there's all the usual marital stuff, you know, two careers, two kids, two work shifts, constant stress. We don't see each other much. And he has guns all over the house, which freaks me out. And I don't always like his meals or his house or his values, or the way he tries to control every little thing, and I'm sure Dan has a list like that too. But I doubt he'll tell you. He's no whiner, I'll give him that."

The counselor puts the folder on her desk and aligns it with her desktop Zen garden. "Next time, I'll see both of you together."

Melissa looks down at the beige Berber carpet as she goes out to the waiting room, feeling as if she has just confessed to a crime. As Dan goes in she sits stiffly in one of the low-backed chairs lined up on either side of the narrow room. She lets her thoughts go. Because the room is empty, she lets them show. She glowers when she thinks of Dan, who says nothing and presumes everything, and clenches her jaw when she thinks of his therapeutic ambush, which is proof that he is so unable to communicate that she should leave him.

Melissa paces to a tall bookshelf at the far end of the room next to a window. She shakes her hands to release her tension, and then takes a blue sugarless candy from a bowl beside a row of books by Jung. She unwraps the candy and bites it. Her teeth hurt immediately, triggering a small regret that expands into a lifetime of regret. She regrets holding back her indecision, ingratitude, and avoidant, adulterous thoughts, but would regret it more if she hurt Dan or gave up the chance to change.

She shouldn't tell anyone what she was thinking that morning after Dan clutched her sweaty back in an agony of ecstasy, and she rolled sadly onto her back, and he said casually, "You've never done that."

"Done what?"

"That thing you did with your—it was—"

"You mean when you were barely inside?"

Dan sighs and nods. His expression is unreadable.

"You didn't like me being on top, did you?"

"You can do that whenever you want," he says condescendingly, with a peck on the cheek.

This time it was Dan who hopped out of bed and took a shower, and Melissa who turned on her side to brood. She still regrets taking the trouble to be on top. She regrets making love with Dan the way she made love with John, because now she is in for a double dose of regret at losing one and never knowing the other.

She regrets her nighttime fantasies of John, and regrets that those fantasies are her only source of partnership. Most of all, she regrets the price she pays for it, which is that she aches for John all the time now, especially during sex with Dan, and in the afterglow. She could tell the counselor all of this, but would regret it, and would regret her regret. Melissa goes to the window and puts her hands on the sill, trying not to look at a forlorn ficus struggling for life in the corner. She presses her forehead against the window glass. *It's okay. Not everything need be felt or said. And everything is beyond my control.*

4

Crux

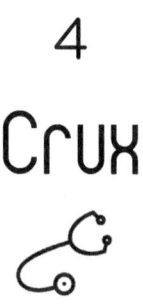

Sarah sits in *virasana* in the new studio, waiting for the trainees to set out their mats for the afternoon session. Her thoughts wander back to last week's reunion in Chicago, and return to Colorado as a young man in white prepares to teach. He stands at the front in a loose shirt and matching pants, rotating his shoulders one hundred eighty degrees to the right, and then to the left. He slides his ribcage fluidly from side to side and circles it around the brim of his pelvis as if willing his spine to liquefy. He bobs his head from side to side, and front to back, his face glowing as if nothing could give him greater pleasure.

The young man sits in lotus position, picks up a hand-held harmonium, and begins to play and sing a *shruti* with sweet devotion. Sarah understands only a few of the words, but can easily enter his feelings of loving wonder. She is enjoying the Rocky Mountains, Zun-Eye Ashram, and her fellow trainees, but it is this teacher who truly captivates her. He is Orpheus enchanting the gods of the underworld, Lemminkäinen luring the moon into a tree, and Bridget opening the door between the worlds to show the bards what lies beyond.

"Take a minute to feel your energy," he says in a reedy voice. "Look around inside your body. Find out if it needs anything." He lets his head fall forward, circles it left and right, and closes his eyes. He says lightly, "You have a type-A personality, and that's okay, that's just the way you are. That's what you work with."

Laughter ripples through the room, settling the high, bright energy of the thirty or so yogis lined up in rows like seagulls facing an onshore breeze. The teacher begins the *asanas* like a maestro of the winds. His students are like birds, first standing, then stretching, then soaring, and then diving. Sarah gives herself up to the symphony of energy that they create, which carries them above the confines of gravity and solidity the way poetry transcends the limits of prose.

Sarah can see that the teacher has entered a universe she can only imagine, a place so rarified that she will have to leave everything behind if she is to join him there. She will have to purify the bad karma imprinted by years of following spurious orders. She will meditate in the Goddess room after class. When she is finished with all of her wasted years, she will be ready to follow her teacher to his Shangri-La.

During *savasannah*, when the students relax after the exertions of class, Sarah recalls her college years and smiles. Her professors prepared her for this. Through the brute force of their arduous homework, she developed powers of attention and concentration to which she is now able to add powers of mental relaxation and devotion. She is blessed. Someday she will be even more blessed through the transformation of all of her life experiences into compassion and other redemptive qualities of being and doing.

When Sarah rolls up her thin, blue mat, she joins the line of trainees who are filing out in silence, shelving their gear. They exit one by one into the alpine landscape that is like a constellation of stars that fell to earth as glistening, snow-clad peaks. Above the trainees' heads, the thin air attenuates into ether, inviting them to be bold enough to penetrate the sky's breath with their spirits. Around them, wilderness offers its unlimited possibilities. Sarah goes to the bunkroom to put on winter gear, and then heads east into open forest on a trough of packed snow that obscures a footpath of gravel and railroad ties. Sarah's footsteps keep time for the wind gusts that sweep over the earthen dam and up the uneven valley to tousle the icy evergreens.

In a clearing near a light gray cliff, Sarah approaches a tiny, peak-roofed cabin and enters its pine-paneled vestibule. Her steamy exhalations paint the air white as she stamps her feet to knock off the snow. She stokes the wood stove and lights it, and when the room is warm, takes off her coat and boots to step into the glass-walled, white-carpeted shrine room that is dedicated to the Goddess. She kneels before a wooden barrier that encloses a row of gilded statues, the largest of which is a life-sized, four-armed Shakti. The sidewalls display mandalas and *thangkas* and an intricate poster of a wrathful blue deity.

Still attuned to sacred time and space, Sarah sits in half lotus, presses her palms together, and gives thanks for the protection of this community, its shrine, and its intention to touch the Divine. She sends a blessing to the young gossip who wrote in her journals, to April, Alan, Doug, Melissa, and John. She sets her intention to purify her karma and polish the mirror of her heart until she can see nirvana in her college years in Hyde Park, where the wheel of life seemed to spin out of control.

After a time, Sarah becomes aware that while the spirit of this place is a joy that she would take to heart, and while it is weakening old harmful patterns of being and doing, it is not weakening her connection to Doug, and she does not want it to weaken her bonds to Melissa and John, or to Patricia or her family. The life here has much to offer, but when her course is done, and she returns to Melissa's home for a brief stay, Sarah will have to answer the questions that life poses by crafting an adult purpose that will enable her to do meaningful work in the world. She can't imagine what that karma yoga will be, or even how to discover it. She can only listen, look, pay attention, and look for a chance to spend her time on earth well.

 When Dan returns from a private meeting with the marriage counselor, he is grave and silent. He barely looks at Melissa during the hour it takes to make dinner. Then he sends the boys outside and leads her into the family room, plumps up the sofa cushions, and puts a box of chocolates on the end table. She sits down and waits, puzzled. After a while, she hears the coffee maker. She hops up, smiles to herself, and goes to sit on a stool at the kitchen island. "Dan, I appreciate your being sweet to me, but shouldn't we talk?"

Dan rattles the utensils in the drawer below the microwave. He scoops the foam out of his plunger pot. His breath snorts in and out through his nose. As he draws a heart in the foam, Melissa's composure cracks. *How can I give up the love of my life for this man, who can't even master enough automatic speech to ask if I had a nice day?* "Dan, talk to me?"

Dan turns away again and leans against the far counter. His back begins to shake. Slowly, Melissa realizes that he is sobbing. Her mind goes numb. She goes to his side and pulls his arm gently. He turns and hugs her tightly. After a while, he relaxes into her embrace.

"I know, Dan, I know. We do our best, but we don't mesh. We don't have enough strengths between us to make a solid couple."

Dan tenses again. He squeezes the breath out of her as he says, "We did until—doesn't all this mean anything to you?"

"The house would be fine without me."

"How could it be fine without you?"

"You could get a younger woman with no career who lives for you. She could do what I do and some of what you do, too. You're a very desirable guy."

Dan makes a choking sound.

Melissa risks levity. "I mean it. You're a homemaker's dream. You're great in bed, you ignore your parents, and you're gone a lot."

Dan shakes his head. He grunts bitterly.

"I'm sorry. That was lame. But we have to find the humor in all this. I mean—I obviously don't have what you need and vice versa."

"You say all these things. Why? What do you expect?"

"I don't—I don't know. Love? Comfort? Acceptance? Support?"

"You have responsibilities!"

"In case you haven't noticed, I've been meeting them for years. And you never express gratitute or praise."

"We need you."

"No you don't. You need a maid, or a housekeeper. Not me. I could love you better if I had someone to care for my soul, and my spirit, or who would do self-care with me."

"I work hard! I provide!"

"Yes. And you're great fun in the outdoors. We're good friends."

"I'm your husband. You're my wife," Dan says plaintively.

Melissa sighs deeply. She can see it now. Dan's inner child has been in charge of their lives since they met. He is helpless, passive, persecuted. No matter what happens to her, he is the victim and it is her fault. She does not know how to partner someone who punishes her for being sick, or who attacks her for having aspirations and values that he did not choose for her. She took off the kid gloves and put on the oven mitts a long time ago.

"I want you to stay," Dan says. "I want you to know that without my having to make a case like a lawyer."

She sighs again and says gently, "I'm not a mind reader. I share what's going on, ask for what I need, and you say and do nothing. I've never seen you express an idea or have a conversation. I've tried everything to have a meeting of the minds and it's never happened."

"Melissa!"

Melissa becomes aware that she is panting and trembling, and that Dan is trying, once again, to quash her feelings with resentment. Melissa pulls her feelings in and down, as if to stuff them under her feet where they will be no trouble to anyone. But this time it doesn't work. She is standing on a geyser made of two decades of disregarded feelings. Her embrace becomes as reluctant and hostile as his. She hisses, "I intend to cure myself in spite of your stonewalling and contempt."

"I always try to help you!" he declares innocently.

She laughs sardonically. He has no insight, no perspective. He is her least competent child. He will be the last to know that he hates her.

"You can't leave!" he commands. "Promise you won't."

Melissa takes a deep and ragged sigh. She begins to cry.

"Promise you won't leave us!" he shouts.

Melissa hears a note of anguish inside Dan's rage. The house of habits they built together was founded on love, but was poorly designed. It is disintegrating, and Melissa doubts that she and Dan can rehabilitate it. She dreams of abandoning its dead weight and starting afresh, hopefully with a partner whose love is strong enough to support a wife.

Eric's face appears for a moment in the doorway. When Melissa sees it she feels ashamed, but this time she responds differently. She fights back. "If you keep on like this, I will leave! I don't want to hurt you or the boys, but I feel crushed. I want support. I need support. I insist that the people I live with be on my side. Or I will live on my own."

"I can change."

"Anyone can, and you will. One way or another."

Doug has finally persuaded Sarah to meet him in San Francisco. He used the aftermath of the reunion as a pretext, but now is truly worried about John, who seems to be going to pieces, and about Melissa, who will have no help at all if John tanks. Doug is so preoccupied by that situation that he passes the window of Café de Lucchi and has to go back up Columbus Avenue to look inside. There she is, sitting on the banquette at the back wall, sipping a cappuccino.

Damn! The minute he sees her he wants her and only her, and not just for the sex. Doug and his wife use terms like emotion and spirituality to make snide jokes. But there sits Sarah, emotionally and spiritually alive, beautiful, smart, bold, and positively glowing with a bandwidth that takes his breath away. He can't see the utter disregard for practicality and material prudence that scares the bejesus out of him and fuels his fears for John and Melissa, who probably live paycheck to paycheck. Sooner or later this recklessness of hers will get under his skin and he will start taking it out on her, but right now he pushes all that aside and thanks his lucky stars that she said yes.

Doug goes in, orders a latte, and takes a seat opposite Sarah at the blond wood table. He tries not to look at the tormented black and blue art on the back wall above her head, which threatens to trigger a bad word. John and Velasquez have been wearing him out. He has no game. He doesn't even have a direction. Once again, he opts for following his gut.

Sarah folds her hands primly on the rumpled napkin in her lap and silently invites him to enter her contentment. She asks placidly, "How are you?"

"I'm worried about John. And Missy."

"Me too. I'm glad you wanted to meet."

"I'm worried about me, too. I could suck your breasts like a baby."

Sarah's mouth opens and her eyebrows go up, but her equanimity holds. "Is it Christy? The sexual issue?"

Doug shakes his head. "She's happy with her woman friends."

"Is it us?"

"No! She's glad my … tastes don't bother you." He sighs. "They are bothering me. I'd like to try something new."

"I'd like that, too." She waits to see if he wants to talk about whatever it is that's bothering him.

He tosses back his coffee drink and with a deep sigh begins, "About the condo…."

When he stalls, Sarah says, "Before you go on, let me tell you that I already promised Patricia I'd become her business partner."

"Whew! I invested some of Christy's money without telling her in a client who turns out to be more manic than Ted Turner."

"Oh, my!"

"Yeah. So I'm in trouble with Christy, and I don't have the liquid assets I thought I would."

"Serendipity is our friend. I'm learning so much from Patricia that I want to stay in the trailer as long as I can."

"Better you than me."

"Yes, exactly. So what shall we do today?"

Doug stretches out his legs with a contented sigh. "I do want to invest in Napa when I have the chance. How about we walk a mile, and catch a ferry?"

"You didn't drive the Rover?" Sarah asks incredulously.

Doug is pleased to have surprised her. "Nope. I wanted to try this European style."

"You mean cold and cramped but cultured?"

Doug flashes her a half smile. "I mean public transit."

Sarah laughs. "Melissa said you hadn't changed a bit, but I think you have."

They exit the midmorning quiet of the café and plunge into the breeze that is rushing over the noisy street. Sarah tips her head back and drinks in the sunshine and mild air. Doug holds his hand at the small of her back. His touch is tender and seductive now, and the space between them is pregnant with promise.

By the time they reach the Embarcadero, however, they are mocking the tourists and tourist traps of Fisherman's Terminal. When she notices this she puts her finger to his lips and says, "Shh! Let's try silence."

This was not Doug's idea. He doesn't like it. He makes faces and wisecracks, but by the time they are standing at the stern of the gently heaving ferry boat, watching the city recede, he is gazing happily at the skinny pyramid of the TransAm Building, the rust-belt wreck of Alcatraz Island, and the ochre span of the Golden Gate Bridge. Sarah puts her head on his shoulder and relaxes into his bulk. He kisses her forehead, pulling her skin like a child sucking a lemon through a peppermint stick.

After the ferry docks at Vallejo, and they have walked to the front of the terminal, Doug mimes unzipping his lips and says, "We'll catch the shuttle here, and the train in town."

"We're taking a train? Where?"

"Up and down Napa. They'll give us lunch and a tour of an Estate, one that grows organic and biodynamic grapes."

"Ooooh! I feel like Persephone leaving the underworld for the warmth of spring!"

When the shuttle drops them at the depot, they gather around the railcar to listen to a conductor with a huge waxed moustache. Doug hands her up the steep steps, and ushers her to reserved seats at an east-facing window. He wonders, *Why am I here? Sex? Luxury? Addiction? Unspoken hopes? Love? Passion?*

The train clears the town, and the waiters bring their pre-ordered lunches.

They stare out of the window at the vineyards, which remind Sarah of the homemade special effects in an avant-garde film. Above, gad-about clouds meld and diverge like froth on a cheese tub. Below, mounds of mustard flowers sway like clusters of jewel lights. Armatures of barren vines glisten like tinsel in a spotlight. In the distance, mountains of crinkled brown napkins hide a watercolor horizon. As the train passes a stand of junipers, though, she spots a trailer and a sun-ravaged worker walking toward a sheep who is browsing at a clump of mustard. This seeming playground is a homey place, with local tasks and particular challenges.

"It's beautiful here," she says.

"You don't mind the clouds this time of year?"

"It's like a greenhouse after Cayuga." Sarah pokes her fork into her salad, sighs, and says, "It's a good thing the condo plan fell through. There are a lot of yoga teachers here already."

Doug raises an eyebrow. "Since when do you do market research?"

"You can tell by the women behind you. They have beautiful posture. Anywhere people have time and money—or simply the vanity or fear that fuels wellness—they will support yoga teachers."

"They don't come up to your standard - or to Christy's."

"I like your taste."

They lunch like two friends who keep a certain distance by talking about nothing important. Sarah expects a casual jaunt followed by consummation of desire, and is content. But when they leave the train for the winery tour, she sees that Doug is serious.

He threads his way through his fellow passengers to shadow the tour guide, and at the end, when they are standing in a field beside the Chateau, Doug asks questions that reflect a detailed knowledge of the Valley and its local politics. As they walk back to the train stop, he leans down to gather a pinch of soil, and sniff it.

"You're becoming a connoisseur of dirt?"

"I want to buy a little vineyard, get my hands dirty. Nothing fancy. Just a hobby, maybe 5000 bottles a year."

"Look up there, then," Sarah says, pointing up the hill to a field worker who is wearing a mask and protective clothing as he sprays the vines in the vineyard above.

Doug does a double take. "Geez Louise." He lopes back to the stragglers of their tour group, collars the guide, and asks, "What's with that?"

"Ah. Well, the neighboring vintners are terrified by the fact that we don't use the usual toxic chemicals. They think the pests will get established here and kill their vines."

"Is that possible?"

"Anything's possible."

"Like people who drink their wine might get sick from the toxins?"

The guide shrugs.

Doug whistles. "Money sure can be stupid."

"And we can be its tools," Sarah says pointedly.

Back on the train, Sarah and Doug sit in silence. The boundary between the sprayed vines and the organic ones haunts him, not least because the spraying was uphill and he is uncomfortably aware that the poisons will be washed downhill. They probably never stay where they're put and never behave as expected. The pluses and minuses of investing—or living—on either side of that boundary go from black to gray and seem to swim away. He can't believe that the poisons are harmless—Christy and her cancer fears have persuaded him of that.

Why aren't locals—or wine lovers—getting sick? Is the effect so insidious that it blends into the background? Or do they hold their wine, poisons and all? *Oh my God! Doctors don't believe in any of that!* They may not see it even when it's happening to them. He seems to feel the floor fall from beneath him. He feels like Harold Lloyd sitting on a train track watching Buster Keaton drive the train away; this feeling of being in an old silent film keeps him from sounding an alarm.

Doug asks Sarah pointedly, "What does Missy eat?"

"Cheap food. The junk with sugar and salt that kids like and that you can pop in the microwave. Unless she's at a restaurant."

"Shit!"

"What?"

"If a guy has to wear a hazmat suit to spray chemicals on grapes, how good can it be for you to drink them, or eat them?"

Very slowly, Sarah begins to see what he is suggesting.

Doug continues, "Most of those chemicals started as agents of biological warfare, and now there are natural ones too."

"Natural?"

"You know, made by plants and animals."

"To protect themselves."

"Nature ain't a love-in."

"Not all of it. Not always."

"Not in human hands," Doug says.

Sarah stares open-mouthed out of his window and says, "Wow. I am become Shiva. He's the creator and destroyer god of Hinduism—That's what Oppenheimer said after seeing the first nuclear test. Think of the implications of poisoning the food supply."

"I am. I've got a crazy organic food producer on the one hand and poisoned terroir that I'm investing in, or was planning to, on the other. Rock and a hard place, that's what I've got. Expensive food that doesn't sell and poisonous food that goes. I *hate* that."

"That's why I can't stay away from you. You see things the way they really are. That's very hard for most of us," Sarah says.

"Except Missy."

"Who's a pessimist."

Doug is quiet for a while, and then, as they roll into the terminal, says, "So it's not because I'm a studmuffin? Or for the perks?"

"I enjoy them. But I don't love them the way I love—and crave—you."

"You were the one who saved me from a bad investment. I should love you."

"But?"

"The less you brag the more you tell the truth."

Sarah raises an eyebrow.

Doug flashes her his shitty grin and then, averting his eyes to the scenery, unable to look at her as he speaks seriously, says, "I hope you like me like I like you because I'm going to stick to you like glue until I die."

John is immersed in the inchoate nothingness that Melissa calls *ayin* and translates from the Hebrew as the ultimate source of all creation that Buddhists call emptiness. He is relieved to finally be here, in the place from which all new constructs arise. He is content. He becomes aware, in the gradual way that dawn arrives in the far north, that it is too dark to see. The nothingness seems to be coalescing around him.

He reaches out to it and finds the soft surface of a bulbous blob. It is his body. Perhaps he is a bunch of grapes. Yes, that must be it. But he did not expect this. He struggles to comprehend his body. He has it! He is a folded immunoglobulin that is circulating in search of a receptor. He is relieved. He is once again content.

His ease ends abruptly when he feels a painful blow to his belly. He tries to raise his head and see what has happened, but he can't move. He must be anesthetized.

This is not what he expected. Something is wrong. Anxiety creeps up his scalp like rising water.

After a mighty struggle, he raises his head and sees his abdomen cut away. He is holding a bloody knife in his hand! He must have cut into his own abdominal wall! Why would he do such a thing? He feels deeply alarmed. He is glad when Leon leans over him. Leon shouts profanely for help as he tries to cauterize John's bleeders. There are too many. John will die. He wants to explain that he did what he did for doctors and patients everywhere. He wants to speak before it is too late, but he can't make a sound. He will die without being heard.

John sits bolt upright. He is sweating and panting and confused. He reaches for Laurel in the bed beside him but his hand lurches into a void. Something falls with a high-pitched thud. He does not know what floor makes that sound. He spies a high rectangle of faint light on his left and another on his right, and realizes that he is on the basement sofa between the high casement window and its reflection in the television screen. He has had a nightmare.

Is this what it's like to find new knowledge? To awaken step-by-step from a nightmare?

Yes. The nightmare of Melissa's illness is only a warning flare discharged across the leaky boat of his life. Cracking her case will come at a cost that is proportional to his blind spots, and his success will only awaken them into a new nightmare. But this is exactly what he signed up for: to protect his species from the hazards they do not see by discovering the truth. The rest is up to them.

John tells himself he should take this realization in stride, but his back is damp, his throat is raw, and his morbid feelings are sticking like cobwebs. He turns on the light and sees the folded top of Tiffany's music stand lying on the carpet beside him. He picks it up and feels its hard edge, seeing why it made him think of a knife, and how he came to be wrestling with it.

John stands and begins to pace back and forth in front of the entertainment unit, suppressing an urge to go upstairs and crawl into bed with Laurel, or with one of the kids. He prefers to sleep here, where he can get up and work, or lie awake, or give himself up to vivid sexual dreams of Melissa that end in climax and sleepy oblivion. If only he could return to the September reunion! At least he can email Melissa. He turns off the light and feels his way up the basement stairs and on to his study, where he sits down in front of the computer and switches it on.

Its beeping and its blue glow offer cold comfort, like the days of late autumn melting into winter darkness. John loves the contemplative feel of fall, though this year it is shadowed by a creeping sense of loss. He thinks back to the warm bed of marriage and ahead to an ever-increasing loss of the innocence and basic trust that come of self-delusion. John resists this by stoking the fire of his virtual affair, which is already blazing.

Get some sleep while I write this, John whispers to Melissa.

In the last email, she asked him for his sabbatical plans. John leans back in his swivel chair and crosses his arms. A car races up the street outside. The pile of manuscripts at his elbow that reminds him of reviews he has yet to do seems to grow in height and weight. He stretches out his legs and folds his hands behind his head.

He reaches into the bottom desk drawer, where he now keeps his exercise clothes, portable CD player, and CDs. He is moving into the study bit by bit, his ties and shoes in the closet, his flashlight on a bottom bookshelf. Soon he will move his LPs up from the basement, but for now he is content to pop a Stevie Wonder CD into the player and put on the headphones. In a minute, he pops it out. His sleepy brain is buzzed rather than lifted by joy. He switches to Coltrane's *Blue* and sits back to ponder. In a minute, he pops that out too; it weighs down his mood like rocks in the pockets. He pops in Miles Davis' *Kind of Blue*. That one is exactly right, not least because he and Melissa made love to it. He allows his body a minute of freedom and then takes off the headphones and puts his fingers to the keys.

Melissa asked for details. He tries to think of some. John snorts in frustration. He knows human beings inside and out, and can care for their needs, but does not know himself or his plans. He wills the blank screen to yield, in vain. He gets up and goes to the kitchen to heat the coffee he left in the pot last night. When he stares at the red on light on the coffee machine, and registers its stale, bitter aroma, he remembers staring at machines like this back in medical school, when working on the wards that burned away his youth and his freedom. As he sloshes the stale coffee into a huge ceramic mug, he remembers the coffee in the doctor's room on the General Medicine ward. He drank it from chewy, too-small Styrofoam cups, took bites of them after, and spit the bites into a plastic-lined metal trash can. That memory unlocks the others, including the night when he gave up on love.

John grabs his throat. His mouth opens to emit a dry sob. He lets his head fall and stares at his feet. Melissa has brought him to a reckoning with his young self. He never grieved for that boy, or forgave him. That boy is the unacknowledged, poorly adapted self that he never knew and can't release.

John feels his way back to the basement, where he lies down and pulls the covers up to his chin. He stares at the square of gray light on the wall. He peels layers of memory from the walls of his mind. They no longer cohere. He is no longer sure who he is, why he is the way he is, or what he should be doing or where and when to do it.

Missy was right. He is at the top of the hill and has nothing left to summit. He is lost, has nowhere to go, and must make sense of his life. Doug was right, too: What is the point of all this effort if it only prepares him to scapegoat his true love? He must solve her mystery to make good on all that has come before. He must improvise.

5

Crash

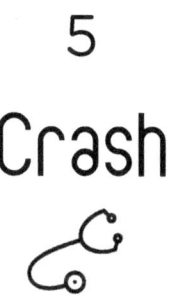

It begins to seem that John's habits—those steady servo mechanisms that support the status quo in the face of every evidence that it is going straight to hell—will contain his reasonable doubts and keep him moving blindly forward. Doug and Sarah even begin to speak of his mid-life crisis in the past tense. And then, one day—the day of the final blizzard of the season—John is overcome by the pointlessness of his precious career.

This morning, after taking his monthly slog through the Departmental budget with a frazzled administrator, he goes to the fitness center to freshen his mind for the brown bag lunch meeting, where the research fellows will report their progress.

John slings his sports bag on his shoulder and imagines that he is Cassius Clay, who became Mohammad Ali, and once had coffee at Jerome's. John trots down the stairs, rapping his knuckles together like The Greatest bumping his gloves on the way to the arena. In the shiny echo chamber of the locker room, John changes into running shorts, a T-shirt reading "North American Association for the Study of Obesity," and crew socks that cover his balding shins. He pushes through the swinging doors into the noisy, glass-walled equipment room like Eric Liddell entering the Olympic oval.

John takes a vacant treadmill with a television monitor and a view of Lake Michigan. He sets the incline and speed higher than usual and runs until his waistband is clammy and his lower back burns. He distracts himself by looking out at the street below, which is bare but for patches of black ice, and nodding to people he knows, like the graying Urologist who climbs endless stationary stairs, the three-hundred-pound pharmacy assistant who struggles to walk, the nurse who does tentative post-partum leg lifts, and the physical therapist who stares at her svelte body in the mirror while sculpting her arms with colorful free weights.

John's race to nowhere pulls energy from his mind to his muscles. He relaxes into the peak experience that is the most grounded part of his workday. When the burn begins to bother him, John looks at the television, but is bored by the lineup of freak tragedies that pass as news and that set up anti-depressant ads. After a few minutes, he notices the news program cut to a commercial showing a slim, handsome young man eating fast food that drips with grease as his friends laugh and dance and fill themselves to the brim for less money than it takes to buy candy at the movies.

John smiles a half-smile at the commercial, which omits unpleasant facts about food, glosses over basic questions about needs and wants, and riffs on the news program's message that daily life is a set up for despair, self-pity, and desire that can be dispelled by consumption. In spite of the fact that he is looking right into the producer's adrenaline-addled mind, John feels wistful for a fantasy world in which eating is cheap fun. He feels an urge to run right into the box so as to live both of its lies—the menacing one that life is a bed of nails, and the shiny one that promises a consumerist lift from misery to happiness.

Suddenly John becomes aware that his ass cheeks are falling and his balls are sagging. He sees everything that commercials edit out of life and that his mind edits out of his life story, which is everything that contradicts notions about medical progress, middle class success, and miracles of technology. He hears his usual voiceover of rationalizations, excuses, and justifications. At the same time, his subconscious mind switches on like a ghetto blaster abusing the back of a bus. The sound overwhelms him.

John hears porky gluttons snorting; clotheshorses whining; lovers gasping as their partners' genitals disappear into folds of fat. He hears hogs squealing at the slaughter; fat-mongers howling; profit-takers cackling; animal lovers sobbing; teeth grinding; throats gulping; bowels bubbling; and the sound of every toilet in Chicago flushing simultaneously. The experience expands to his other senses. He smells blood-splattered abattoirs, spoilt meat, sour vomit, flatus, and guts cut open on the operating table. He feels pork rinds smearing his fingers; a lump of lard gagging his gullet; reflux burning his chest; and stool blocking his bowels.

John's mind has broken free of its well-crafted frame. Everything he suppressed or repressed or denied is spurting out of his id and gathering into a anti-consumerist ghoul that wears a silent Edvard Munch Scream and shouts, *Stop stuffing your craw!* The specter eats through the ad John has been living in for as long as he can remember, and spits out several pieces of the gyroscope that has been sustaining his worldview.

John's carefully cultivated optimism collapses. Everything he saw as good or neutral now looks bad. His life story is a tense, tedious, bone grinding, blood draining, ineffectual, and inadvertent counter advertising campaign. He pursues million-dollar decoy-grants while his patients glut themselves on memes and foodstuffs unfit for pigs. He spent his prime and a pile of public money pursuing a fat-melting pill that would only enable the dark side of the status quo. Outside his frame, in the real world of gluttony and sloth, science is beside the point.

John laughs wildly. His co-workers stare askance. Their silent censure is a cold slap to his ego. He sucks in his lips and resumes his run. He tries to outrun his vision. He can't. He can see that he is running in place. He increases the incline all the way to pull the blood from his brain and blot out the vision. It doesn't work. He can't escape.

John lets go. He gives his vision free rein. His blind spots disappear. His filter appears. He sees that it is designed to hide his compulsive conformity, self-brainwashing, wishful thinking, excuses, and self-justification. The loss leaves him with nothing to lean on and no way to get his bearings. For a minute, his life is like an M.C. Escher drawing in which foreground becomes background. Then the foreground resolves into a cage. He becomes the rat running on the wheel.

The old story of his life, which was made of moments of care and cure and the saving of young lives, was edited together from years of senseless drudgery that are still taking up space on the server of his memory. He can't bear to look at the endless hours he spent watching while his patients inflated themselves like piles of tires waiting to blow out. It reminds him of the first time he saw a landfill, and realized that his trash didn't just disappear. *I'm all motion and no action! If I drop everything I've been working on, the world will lose nothing and I'll be able to do what matters!*

John can't stand it anymore. He jumps off the treadmill, pauses in the locker room to throw on a sweat suit, and runs all the way outside and north on the wide sidewalks. He passes pedestrians leaning into the wind like skaters, threads the dank underpass at Lake Shore Drive, crosses the frosted sands of Oak Street beach, and pounds up the treed path along the water's edge. He runs eagerly into the pain of the icy lake breeze, fleeing a land of shadows for a future that may be filled with hope or despair.

Insight sticks to John like an oil slick. He used to admire and covet it, but now that he has it he would like to fob it off on some unsuspecting stranger. He would like to go blissfully back into the waking sleep in which he blames his malaise on a bad marriage and escapes into the love of his life. Neither divorce nor love can dispel this dark vision, though, which is his, and is in him and of him. He wonders if Melissa can see it too, and whether it drives her conscience. He will ask her. He will call as soon as he can. *Thank God for you, Missy! With you I can do anything. I hope I can do as much for you.*

John stops and leans forward, panting, his hands propped on his bent knees. He is halfway to Belmont Harbor without a pager or a penny. Snow is falling heavily on the cement of the city, muffling traffic noise and converting the cement path into a sea of slush. John realizes that he must be late for his noon meeting. A year ago, a lapse like that would have filled him with angry shame. Now he accepts it as inevitable. John summons his strength and lopes back to the hospital, ignoring his bone deep chill, and his sliding, slipping feet.

When John sees his office window come into view, he feels nothing in particular. His cage is not the office, the job, or the building. It is the mindset he carries around like a backpack that he can't see because it is behind him. He can feel it, though. It will take every particle of his patience to wear it until he can shed it without harming the people who depend on him. *I have to change now, but I can't let it show!*

When he reaches the service entrance of the hospital, John's vanity rallies. He leaves a series of wet prints on the floor like a dotted arrow pointing to his office. People smile knowingly and talk about the weather. He is beginning to hope that his lapse escaped notice until he hurries through his outer office and hears Evetia announce sharply, "I canceled your afternoon appointments."

"Oh," he says sheepishly. "Thanks. I, uh, got caught out in it."

He retreats to his inner office and sits down to scan his messages for signs of trouble. He finds none. He feels tentative relief. *Maybe I've ducked the backlash.*

"Who you think you fooling?" demands Evetia harshly. "Look at you! You a mess!"

John turns toward his angry-eyed keeper. She closes the door and sits on the edge of one of the University of Chicago chairs facing his desk. She wraps her long-nailed, spidery fingers around the armrests as if trying to keep her hands from strangling him. She continues her cool rant. "You want people to believe my lies, you got to tell me what's going on."

Evetia has always adhered to strict formality. She has always called him doctor, taken a seat only when invited, kept a lid on her attitude, and spoken Standard English. Now she is scolding him the way she berates her ten-year-old when he does something wrong at school.

John's first impulse is to feed her a vague cover story. "I'm having problems at home."

Evetia raises her brows, pushes herself to her feet like a reporter with a scoop and a deadline, and bolts for the door. Now that he has revealed his situation thus far, though, he can't seem to stop. "I need a sabbatical, and I need it now, and Laurel won't go."

Evetia whirls around, and lets fly. "Don't you go off on me, now! I got people depend on me. My mother, my sister, my kids. I got to work."

He observes dryly, "You're not the only one."

"You got choices I don't," Evetia retorts.

Evetia will try to keep him in his cage. She will want to handle him the usual way and get the expected results. She will want him to stay steady so she does not have to worry about him in addition to everything else in her life that needs care and attention. Everyone he knows, with the exception of Melissa, will react in this way. He accepts it.

"I'll be sure you have a good position while I'm gone. How'd you like to work for Dr. Jake Breen in Peds? He's a good man."

"I don't want no good man. I want a strong one. That why I work for you."

Clearly, Evetia sees no virtue in vulnerability. John will have to show the flexible tenacity that is the hallmark of strength over time. He says firmly, "I know what I owe you, Evetia. You can count on me. But change is coming, and you may have to work for a nice man for a while."

"Now you scaring me. You scaring me now." Evetia flashes him a crooked smile of collusion. "And don't you leave out of here 'till I get those clothes you left down in that gym."

When Evetia has deposited his clothes on his desk, John abandons his plans to shower, puts on his work clothes and heads for the car. He climbs into the cushioned cocoon of the cold driver's seat, puts on his car gloves, and grips the steering wheel. He puts the key in the ignition. He listens to tires squeal on a lower level. He has no idea where to go or what to do.

John lets his head sink back into the headrest. An hour into his new life, he is exhausted. The patterns he spent years creating and mastering and intensifying became effortless. Without them he is like a train stopped at the end of the tracks. The engine of his habits may be warm and able to overcome his inertia, but there is nothing ahead to support his continuation.

Behind him is the innovative wave front of hope-filled, labor-driven industry that produces the grand technologies at the heart of the hospital, like the new CT and radiation therapy suites, as well as the simpler marvels of ubiquitous wheelchairs, electric beds, intravenous pumps, cardiac monitors, and so on. Gone are wards of patients cared for with gauze and kindness. Here is the hope of unlimited privilege made manifest in mechanization, isolation, disposability, elaboration, and promises of cure that fade into drug dependence. It isn't what it seems. He will have to lay track through unknown terrain.

After an indefinite period that is a near blank, John gets out of the car, grabs his exercise bag and briefcase, and begins to walk. The next thing he knows he is riding up the elevator of the nearby Drake Hotel, a flat key gripped between his fingers. He gets out at his floor and walks along the lavishly carpeted hall like a celebrity who is holing up in rehab. To shake off his furtiveness, John talks himself up. He reminds himself that he stays in hotels like this when he travels on business. Anyone looking at him would take him for a customer paying for gracious privacy. Unfortunately for John, withdrawal sets in before he reaches the room. He can feel his fingers typing his task list the way a former smoker feels a phantom cigarette.

The room's interior is comforting. The conservative constancy of its Queen Anne furniture, forest green drapes, and floral linens promises to anchor his body so that his mind can wander freely. He cooperates with its staid spell by doing things he usually does when checking into a hotel. He lifts his bag onto a caddy, puts his clean things in drawers, and sends dirty ones to the laundry. He calls Evetia to let her know how to reach him. He turns on his pager and puts it under the bedside lamp. Then he decides to break his habits by doing whatever comes into his head.

John grabs a snack from the mini-bar, hops onto the bed, picks up the remote, and flips through the channels of the small television set. As he is popping a second handful of peanuts into his mouth, he freezes. He laughs again, with less edge. He has taken normalcy too far. His mind is running the couch potato program he uses when he sits in the family room with the children. This is the very behavioral loop that has trapped so many of his patients in prisons of fat.

John jumps up and paces back and forth. After a period of near blankness, a memory arises. He is walking a ridge trail between two chasms. To fall either way will mean instant death. He feels the grip of fear and an intense desire for control. He stops in consternation. He walked that Rocky Mountain trail decades ago but never left it. He guided his patients and mentees and family as if the risk of falling was all that mattered. He forgot to lift his eyes from the trail to take in a glimpse of the miracle of creation that is spread out all around.

John reminds himself to do whatever comes into his head. After a brief nothingness, John takes off his clothes and takes a long, steamy, mid-afternoon shower. When he is done he takes the heavy courtesy robe from the closet and puts it on. He cannot remember doing this before. This small innovation heartens him. He sits down in the floral armchair. He waits. He tries to see the unknown future by holding it in front of his mind's eye like a crystal ball, but he cannot formulate a question with the power to raise a vision. He lets his willpower lapse. He waits.

His next impulse is to do something wild. He considers this and laughs. This impulse is a staple of Hollywood scripts, a starting point for tragicomic fantasies, a first step in cautionary tales that date back before the moving image, before limelight, before amphitheaters, and before cave paintings. It is a recipe for regret. He lets it go. He wants to break with the past as smoothly as he can. *First, do no harm.*

John's patience is broken by a tingle of desperation that makes his gut feel like a set of vibes. *Do something new, anything!* He jumps up and closes the drapes, turns off the lights and lies down on the bed. He smiles. This is his program for sleep, which is old but necessary. After a pause he gets up, lies on the floor next to the writing desk, and moves his arms and legs if making an angel in the snow. He realizes that this program, too, is old, and recently activated by an airline magazine article about using playfulness to increase productivity.

John balls his fists and drums them on the carpet. He feasts on frustration. *With my education and experience, how will I ever think of something new?* He lies still and waits. His fists relax. *It needn't be new!* He knows how to do this. He knows how to move into the unknown. Research has kept alive his inborn curiosity and honed his skills. His body relaxes. He lets go of anticipating and controlling and reacting and doing. He becomes completely still.

Memories pass before his mind's eye like seeds on the wind. He is a boy in the north woods watching a fish swim over a tannin-stained streambed. He is waiting to play a set at The Hive when the house lights are low and the metal harp is cold in his palm. He is walking by Jackson Park listening to drumming fill the quiet night in Hyde Park. He is hiking in an alpine meadow with a map and a compass. He is atop Long's Peak, exhilarated by the spine of the Rockies. He is making an incision in wrinkled skin stained by yellow-brown Betadine.

He is playing golf with Leon. He is watching Laurel turn away as he enters her. He is listening to her say that she will not leave her life. He is listening to Leon's advice about staying married. He is hearing every vulgar thing Leon ever said about women. Bits and pieces click together into a pattern he recognizes with a flash that is like a diagnosis. Leon has been shtupping Laurel to weaken John. John grunts bitterly. Melissa said he could handle any truth, but he has been a stranger to the truth. His home life is a far bigger sham than he had guessed. It is a farce that makes him ridiculous and makes Laurel pathetic.

John hops up too fast and has to bend over to counter his light-headedness. When he regains his balance he slides into the desk chair and dials. He uses the full force of his powerful will to find the numbers on the phone. *I hate you! I hate you! I hate you both!* John's face contorts with feelings that shift from outrage to revulsion to masochistic triumph. He squeezes the edge of the desk with his free hand and forces regular breaths.

After several rings, Laurel answers.

"Are you happy?"

"John? Is that you?" He notices that his wife is shocked that he would call, and that there is a hint of concern in her hard voice.

"Are you happy with Leon?"

"I thought it was an emergency or I wouldn't have answered."

The hint of concern was for her. She's cut me loose! "Laurel! *Answer* me!"

"Are you happy with her?"

"We had dinner once and we write. We haven't—we don't—"

"Don't you try and dump me! I'll take everything. I've had the best divorce lawyer in Illinois on retainer for a year. If you keep shut until Leon leaves his wife, I'll go easy on you."

"You must know—" John freezes. The bottom falls out of his anger. He feels a stab of pity. Laurel has never been particularly bright or canny. She has no idea that Leon is never going to leave his wife, or that Leon used her to get at her husband. His chest contracts into a dull ache. He can't breathe. He considers and dismisses the possibility of heart disease. "I know what I owe you. You married me for money and children and security. I provided them, and I'll continue to provide them. For your sake as well as for the children."

"And I will continue to do every little thing you can't be bothered to think about. Except one."

His voice scrapes his larynx. "Our plan wasn't enough, was it? We should have taken risks, tried new things." He hears water running and feels a stab of panic. "Who's with the kids?"

"They're with me after school and then with my parents. As usual. As you should know."

"I'm not coming home for a while. You can call Evetia if you need me."

John hangs up numbly. He goes to the curtains and opens them. He blinks away a stab of bright light. Outside, the wind is shredding the clouds to make way for the sun's rays. Below, office workers in winter coats dodge dawdling window shoppers. He imagines that he hears the sounds of tires splashing up the busy, slushy street. Judging by the shadows cast by the stoplights, it is still mid-afternoon.

John puts on dry exercise clothes and running shoes. He jogs downstairs, across the flower-carpeted lobby, and out through the shiny, brass wrapped front doors onto the sidewalk of East Walton Place. Multicolored hotel flags ruffle in the cold wind, drowning out the pinging of an idling tour bus. Tourists chatter as they wait for their bus driver to worm their bags into its open luggage compartment. The doorman raises his voice and razzes a regular who is approaching from Michigan Avenue, his tie flapping behind like a streamer.

John jogs to Michigan Avenue, turns, and window shops his way to the Water Tower monument, where he stops beside a lone derelict to look up at the tiny stone relic. He sees the unedited history of Chicago spinning on its axis. He sees the ancient swamp, the peoples who traveled it in canoes, the great pine forests sucked out of the heartland by the builders of the wooden city that burned in 1871. He sees the immigrants who fled old countries to find work as gandy dancers, slaughterers, bathtub gin bootleggers, gangsters, commodities gamblers, and builders of the metal cages that are reaching up to consume the very sky. He sees people striding purposefully past to take their places in those cages, where the mindless machine of the economy is training them to do rat-tricks for money-chow. *Why don't they wake up and take charge of their lives? Why don't I?*

Suddenly, something pitches John forward. A pain radiates from his back ribs. His leg burns. An angry exclamation claps his ears. "Watch where you're standing!"

John sees a splash of coffee on the leg of his sweat suit and looks up in astonishment. It has been a long time since he was treated roughly and rudely on the street. Several feet away, John spots the angry face of a drug company salesman who frequents the hospital. With him is a man from the office of the Chief of Staff. Shock and embarrassment spread over both men's faces as they realize that the sales rep just shoved and insulted the Chairman of Medicine. John feels the tension of status confusion, and an impulse to reaffirm the hierarchy.

"You may not want to exercise, but you don't have to assault those of us who do," John says with a glib smile.

"I'm so sorry," the rep replies obsequiously, clearly relieved that John has defined the incident as a joke. "Bad day. You okay? That was—can I buy you a coffee?"

John shakes his head, salutes cordially, and jogs away, aware that he has just felt the tenuousness of his place on the ladder of success. He has climbed it long and far enough to know that if he loosens his grip on his rung, peers like Leon will push him off. He pictures himself crashing at the bottom like a misshapen Rumpelstiltskin prop in a school play. He sees his supporters peeling off after him and landing on him like a heap of hand-sewn puppets. He sees a free-for-all as others scramble to take their old places. *That's why we continue as we do. We see the ladder and fear the fall.*

At the next intersection, John turns toward the Lake. The vision spooked him, but he can laugh at it. Walking out of the hospital and into his hotel room was the hard part. It took every bit of his courage to walk away from his responsibilities, even for a day. Everything that happens from now on is a first chance to make good on that bold move. Despite his awareness of risk, John is already more at home in his skin, and more alive than he has been in years. He will be fine if he keeps his mind off

Laurel's indiscretion. He is not ready to think about that yet. It is glowing like a red-hot cast iron skillet on the back burner of his mind. He will have to turn down the heat and wait for it to cool. When he has left for sabbatical he will toss it on the scrap yard of memory and melt it down with the other refuse that is cluttering his mind! He will put it behind him.

John puts his lips together and plays them like a mouth harp. He finds a walking baseline. Before his lab became his refuge, he relied on music to carry him out of fixity and into fluidity. John picks up the pace. Rarefied excitement rises in his mind. He reaches the hotel in minutes and takes the stairs two at a time up to his room, where he flips through the phone book. He finds the listing he wished for. Major Green Music has moved to South Shore, but is still in business. John washes and grooms and darts outside and over to the parking garage to pick up his car. In minutes, he is speeding south.

During the past ten years, he has driven this way only to go to Hyde Park. Now he is driving farther south and back in time past the juke joint called The Hive, where for a few glorious months he played with professional musicians.

Muddy was quite a mentor to many a young musician. He was tough and lascivious and wild and brave and canny. He played like a music surgeon who cut dead tissue from the hearts of listeners so that healthy tissue could grow in its place. He did it with artistry, with transgressions, and with no clear regard for consequences. Muddy is still John's model for breaking with the past, redeeming rage, showing courage, and cultivating the mischief that can bring music to life.

Muddy had stumbled as a husband and father, and yet stayed steady as a mentor. That thought gives John heart. *Stay with me,*

Muddy; take me to music that will play me into the next set of this crazy life.

John notices that he has already passed the grassy expanse of Grant Park; the straightened s-curves of Lake Shore Drive; the Field Museum; the gray Greek columns and greenish glass of the new Soldier Field; and the overpass of black steel at McCormick Place. He exits at South Shore, rolls slowly down the main street, and parks as near as he can to the store. He trots eagerly up the cracked sidewalk to peer at the window display, which is obscured by heavy metal accordion bars. The new and used instruments would suit a lowbrow pawnshop, but if the Major has kept up standards, the inventory in the back will be exceptional.

John's view of the material world shifts like a hologram from dark dystopia to sweet utopia. This cornucopia holds the keys to his personal happiness, and the money he has earned from the desire-crazy economy will buy them for him. When the door closes behind him with a chime, John pauses to stare at the walls, which are covered with reeds and drumsticks and tuning forks and every little thing a musician might want, all locked up behind glass. A coughing fit arouses him from this vision of musical plenitude. John notices an old black man with knobby hands behind the counter. His thin hair is as sheer and white as the stalk of smoke rising from his ashtray. His leonine eyes and wide mouth are surrounded by drooping parentheses of folded, faded skin. He is wearing a green cardigan like Mister Rogers'. John nods. "I want to see the best sax you've got in stock."

The old man raises his eyebrows and runs a deeply skeptical glance from John's toes to his head. He shrugs and goes through a curtain at the back, from which he emerges several minutes later with a shiny saxophone case. He hefts it on to the counter with some difficulty and opens the top to reveal a brass horn that looks to be made of solid gold.

John swallows hard, pulls off his driving gloves, takes off his coat, and lifts the instrument awkwardly. Surprisingly, his hands find their way. He feels the action of the keys and frowns. He looks at the price tag and returns the sax to its black velveteen bed. He smiles crookedly. "I said your best one, not your most expensive one."

"Uh-huh," the man says with a grumpy look. "What you looking for?"

"Mellow, sweet, easy. Something the Bird would have blown."

The old man rolls his eyes. "You just starting lessons?"

"I'd better. It's been almost twenty years." John swallows and rests his hands on the counter.

"Hmph. What you used to play?"

"A student instrument. A Conn I bought from you. The only one I could afford at the time. I had a good harp though. And I used to borrow a ten thousand dollar clarinet. But not often!"

The old man raises his eyebrows and chews his lips. He nods, takes the case to the back, and brings out a case and a plastic bag of reeds. He hands the latter to John. "It been that long, you better use this soft one. Maybe it won't cut your tongue." He hefts the case onto the counter and says, "Try this one first."

John takes a few breaths to open his lungs and freshen his mind. He snaps open the case, puts his hand on the cold bell, and scoops out the body. He puts the reed into the mouthpiece, closes his lips around it, and blows to warm the brass. His hands help to warm the metal.

John closes his eyes, puts his tongue on the reed and tests the mouthpiece. He has no embouchure at all. He lets his hands remember and his mouth keep up as best it can. He plays a slow scale, and then a faster one. His fingers lose their rhythm at higher speeds. He plays fifths and sevenths, and segues into a rusty riff from Coltrane's Blue. His mouth hurts already. He is losing control of his lips. His cheeks puff out. John hears a wheeze and opens his eyes.

The old man is laughing. "You looking like Dizzy, now. You on the wrong instrument."

John stretches his mouth into an O. "What else you got?"

The old man raises his brows but goes to the back and brings out two more cases. John is glad they are alone in the store. He can take his time. He doesn't look at the prices now. He pulls a melody out of the air and plays with volume and timbre. He tries several styles on each of the three instruments, switching reeds as he goes, emptying them of saliva.

"I remember you, now!"

John stares at the old man for a few seconds. "Have I seen you in clinic?"

The old man raises an eyebrow. "You played The Hive with Muddy. You that skinny, skinny little white boy. When you went up on that stage, I thought, that little stick can't make no kind of sound, but you had a big, round sound. Too big, some time. I said to myself, why he whining on that tinny harp when he got some *air*?"

John stares at him in astonishment. "You and I must be the only ones that remember that."

"You don't remember me. Huh-uh. I'm Mr. Cotton. The Major, he died recently, and I mostly putter around here nowadays."

"I'm sorry, I didn't—it's been so long. Well, it's good to see you looking so good."

"Liar! My face bout to drag on the ground. Hah-huh. You want lessons?"

"I'd love to start right away."

"Well, I know a couple of retired players could use work. After you get your chops back, you be okay. You won't waste they time. They don't take beginners, now. Nope. No beginners. So, which one you want?"

John inhales for inspiration. He would be happy with any of the three, but the silvery, custom-made one with several dents captured his fancy. "How much for this one?"

"That depend."

"On what?"

"On what else you buy. You need a harp?"

Later, on the drive home, John feels like a teetotaler who went on a money bender. He was never a big spender. He feels a need to justify the rash extravagance of a hotel stay, a trunk load of instruments and supplies, and an upcoming lesson. He points to Laurel's emeralds, her sexual follies, and her legal bloodlust. John grips the steering wheel and grunts in rage. The back burner of his anger heats up. His cast iron skillet of rage rattles and sputters angry thoughts.

She should have known that she would lose John's respect and interest. *I will never sleep with her again.*

John steadies himself with the thought of playing music. He runs his mind over the instruments in the trunk. He moves his fingers on the steering wheel, walking the pattern of a blues line. He hears a melody that can sing his soul out of its cage and help him find his future. When he gets to the room he will wrap his lips around his new sax and play. When he is played out, which may take hours, he will be calmer, and may be able to put his thoughts in order. *I will need a lawyer. I will need to talk to the Dean!*

By the time John has dashed furtively back to the hotel room with his instruments in his arms, he is calmer and able to think more clearly. In the room, he puts down his instruments, takes a seat at the desk, and fights a wave of nausea. When he picks up the telephone receiver, though, he feels a white light on his right shoulder. It is familiar and reassuring. It fills him with wellbeing. It is Melissa. She used to put her hand there when she stood behind him at his desk in their shared apartment. Back then, he would reach up and put his hand on hers, but now he sits still and concentrates and breathes slowly and deeply. After a few minutes, he is breathing easily. He is feeling loved. As he dials, he thinks, *Stay with me, Missy!*

"Hello?" replies the Dean's voice.

John hears a boy's voice haranguing in the background. He knows the Dean has children, but has never before seen or heard them. John clears his throat. "Laughlin here. Sorry to bother you at home, but I'm calling to give notice. I have some leave coming and I'll start taking it tomorrow. Colin can take over the lab and the Assistant Chair can take the Department with Evetia's help. I'm sorry, but I uh—think it's best if I don't come in again."

The Dean inhales sharply. "Hold on, John. I need to get to my study."

John hears footsteps slap across a floor. He hears a door close, an echo, and a creak. John can see the Dean, a sedentary, older man, sitting on the toilet in his bare feet. John suppresses a smile. He is feeling giddy, and a little lightheaded.

The Dean pants, "Well, John, I've been expecting this call for a long time—"

"I know. I've been off lately, which is why I shouldn't risk coming in—"

"No, no, I mean I've been expecting this call since your first promotion."

"I didn't realize—"

"What I meant to say, John, is we promoted you too quickly. For your own good, I mean. It's been great for us—you're the best Chair we've ever had. The clinicians respect you, the teaching faculty respects you, and the researchers respect you. You know how rare that is. I've never told you, but you've herded all those cats better than any of us could have hoped. But I knew it was risky to ask so much of you, John, and I'm sorry I didn't bring it up earlier."

John can't organize his thoughts to field a reply. The Dean always seemed dissatisfied, always hinted that things could be better. *Was he trying to keep me hungry?*

"You're way overdue for a sabbatical, John. Go now, and take all the time you need. Go abroad, check out the competition, take stock of things, do whatever you need to do to get back in gear. I'll take care of everything at this end. We can huddle in the morning, won't take a minute, and then you can go to the airport if you want."

"I don't know. I don't know if I can—"

"Don't worry about Leon's grab for your lab space. I've got your back." The Dean's voice drops to a whisper, "Just between you and me, he's desperate. Can't handle the research side. And his tactics are, uh, unacceptable. He won't be here when you get back."

John's brain feels numb. The middle of his face is shame-red.

"Look, John, something like this happens to all of us, sooner or later, if we're in this game long enough. It happened to me. You may not remember this, it was before your time, but I had a different wife when I came here from Duke."

John shakes his head until he remembers that the Dean can't see him.

"When I first got here, it was a heady time, and stressful. My first wife resented me for taking her away from her family, and I resented her spoiling my success, and one night I told my troubles to one of the statisticians, and one thing led to another. I left my wife for her, which caused a big scandal. I felt sorry for myself at first, but I gradually came to see I'd set a terrible precedent. It hurt morale in both departments. I vowed to get on top of things before they got out of hand."

John is panting. He reaches for the place on his shoulder where he felt Melissa's hand and tries to recover his sense of wellbeing. *Come back Missy; help me through this scandal!*

"A crisis tests your character, John, but I'm not worried about that." The Dean makes a sound like a low chuckle. "I'm worried you'll find something better. If you do, that's that. But as long as you want your old job, it's yours."

"But—"

"And if you want to step down and devote yourself to your new research program, that's fine too. Your article in Nature, your plan for a new center, that's what we all want. And John, I know this isn't about money, but we can sweeten the deal. I can free up some seed money for that center. Just give me the word and it's done."

" I, uh … I … "

"Call me in three months, John. No sooner. Three months."

"I don't know if I can afford—"

"Full salary and benefits, of course. And travel money. I'll get you a Departmental credit card. You mentioned Italy. Take your family, or your companion."

John's hand clasps his shoulder. *My companion.* They all think he strayed too, or maybe the Dean wants him to think that.

"We can make it six months, or twelve if you need more time. Okay, John? Okay?"

"Okay. Okay, Bruce. Thanks. That's—I don't know what to say—confusing time—"

"Good. Good. I'm sure you'll use that card wisely—for expenses," the Dean adds anxiously.

John smiles. The Dean is known for being tight. "Don't worry. It may not take that long."

"Don't call me before three months. Call me in three. Or six."

John feels cautious gratitude. *Does he really want me back, or is he only buying time?* "Okay. Three months. Thanks. I... uh, I ..."

"Say nothing of it, John. We value your contribution. We're behind you one hundred percent. We'll talk more later, have a heart to heart. In a few months—or more."

John's laugh catches in his throat. He chokes out, "Three. Three months."

6

Create

A phone rings as John drives north in the dark from the Amalfi Coast to Tuscany, where he will learn to work with marmosets in a research lab in Siena, and so use his sabbatical to extend his work to other species. He notices the ringing sound and extricates his flip phone from his jacket pocket and replies tensely, "Hello?"

"John! I'm glad I caught you."

"I have to hang up. I'm due in Siena. I decided to go via the Amalfi coast and there's very little to see but the road is windy. I may have to drive all night!"

Melissa lifts her spoon and strikes it against the edge of a pot on the stove. She is relieved that he is okay, alarmed that he is talking while driving, and appalled that he has no insight about how to care for himself nor any perspective on his workaholism. The tables turn: She is the doctor and he is the patient. She says, "John! You're in Italy!"

"Yes."

"John! Pull over! We have to talk."

"I don't have time!"

"I need your full attention right now. Get off the road. I'll hang on."

John grunts irritably and grudgingly relents. "If you insist."

As John exits the roadway, Melissa holds the phone between her ear and her shoulder, turns off the burner, ladles chili into a bowl, and sits at the counter. She takes up a spoonful of hearty beans and blows on it to cool it.

John comes to a stop, takes a deep breath, and says, "Okay, shoot."

"Look at yourself!" she laughs. "Do you see what you're doing?"

John frowns and says, "Sitting behind the wheel?"

"I mean the way you're living. You're addicted to busy. You're the workhorse who can't stop following the carrot around the millstone. You have to treat that the way you would any addiction."

"But I'm due at the lab in the morning!"

"Call and say you'll be in next week, or the week after. Italians will think you're crazy if you don't take time to enjoy their country. And they'll be right."

"If I don't start I won't have time for you. You choose."

"I choose that you gear down. You'll be of no use to me if you don't take time to think. You can do it. You're not on call now. Nobody is going to die."

"I can't waste time!"

"It isn't wasting time—it's living. That's what you're supposed to be doing."

"I'm no addict!" he says fiercely.

"Prove it."

"How?"

"Sabbatical is a rabbinical word that refers to the sabbath. The purpose is to do the work that you've put off for twenty years at least. The work of contemplating the big, eternal questions of life, like where have I been and where am I going and why. It isn't a sabbatical if you live as you usually do. You'll defeat the whole purpose—which is to stop and think and be and become wise. It's critical when you're burned out; if you don't do it right, you risk wasting the rest of your life. I can get you started. Follow this prescription: get off the road; find a hotel room with a view and a balcony and room service. Go to sleep."

"Missy!" John replies as if speaking to a small child. "I'm here to work."

"I'll give you a daily check list. Do you have paper and a pen?"

John grunts and fumbles in his pockets for paper and a pencil. "Go on."

"Stay in bed as long as you can. When you can't stay in bed any longer, order a meal, take it out onto the balcony, and eat at a leisurely pace. Watch the water—for at least three hours. Count the waves, time them, and estimate their height. Record everything you observe and then draw a detailed picture of what you see. The next day, do the same thing but go to the shore instead of the balcony. The day after, put the drawings in an envelope and send them to me. Then call me. Do you have all that?"

"How can I get anything done that way?"

"Your mission is to transition to sabbatical mode, to break with the past, to study, to renew yourself, to refresh your ideas. It's like Shabbat."

"That's why I want to get to the lab!"

"If you go there you'll do what you always do. You can't deal with the unknown like that. You have to shake things up, form new insights and perspectives, do something original. You'll have to do all of that to help me."

John sighs tensely. "When can I go to the lab?"

"Let's take it one step at a time. Expect it to be the hardest thing you've ever done and you won't be disappointed. And expect it to cost time—and effort."

John sighs deeply. "Sleep does sound good. I do feel exhausted."

"Good! If you sleep for three days straight, so much the better. You'll be fresh and able to get back to being curious and engaged and observant and able to live in real time."

A week later, Melissa is lying on the sofa in the greenhouse addition, tea tray and flip phone beside her on the floor. She is bundled in wool clothing and covered by a thick duvet. She winces in pain and rearranges her legs carefully. She relaxes, but begins to shiver. She lifts a large cup of steaming tea with difficulty and takes small sips. She begins to cry. Her phone rings. She inhales deeply, wipes her tears with her sleeve, and answers, "Hello?"

John picks up a pencil and holds it poised over a pad of lined yellow paper. "So tell me how it started."

Melissa laughs through her tears. Her expression radiates consolation. She sits up carefully and says, "Tell me about the Uffizi! I want to live vicariously."

"Time is too short. Tell me your present medical history."

"What about the drawings?"

"You wanted me to live like an Italian. The drawings will get there when they get there."

Melissa laughs deep in her throat. Speaking to John is easing her pain and lifting her spirits. "Do you want an ordinary history or my systematic observations?"

"Let's start with an ordinary history of the present illness, and then the past medial history and treat your observations as part of our assessment."

"Right-o. I was perfectly well until my first pregnancy, when ..." She tells him the long, slow sequence of symptoms and diagnoses that triggered treatments that added to her problems and made it difficult to detect any pattern in them.

"Occam's razor," John says.

"Exactly! It must be one thing."

"Or a few."

"And it causes a positive review of systems!"

"Symptoms in every organ system?"

"Like syphilis or AIDs."

"An agent of disease that affects everything."

"But not everyone."

"I see the problem."

"It affects all of me. I have gastritis, depression, asthma, signs of auto-immune disease and allergy, and—most of all— problems with every aspect of my nervous system, including the autonomic nerves."

"Huh. If I didn't—if it wasn't you, I'd think you were a malingerer. Or a nut."

Melissa counters, "That's how we react to the unknown as clinicians. And then refer to infectious disease or psychiatry. And if that doesn't work, punishment. If I hadn't been on your side of cases like this it would be hard for me to forgive you, or the system."

John is silent. He begins to breathe heavily. He is not sure what he is feeling. He is not sure what he has been doing in life. After a time he hears himself saying, "This is the reason I went to the U of C for med school. This is the reason I took that independent study in medical detection."

Melissa is shocked to hear John speak as if he believes in

predestination, or in touching eternal time. She waits for him to continue.

John goes on, "I wanted to be ready to grapple with the unknown. I love the lab, I'm having fun here in Siena. But I'm always aware that meeting expectations is no way to advance the field. You need a wild card. You need chance. A chance like this."

Melissa laughs sardonically, and then says, "It'll be worth it to me if you and I can turn it to the good."

"You're my other half. I'll do what I can. Call me when you get a flare-up and we'll talk it through."

"I'd like that. I keep asking myself how the medical system could have failed me so completely—from education to research to clinical care to complex systems to life as a patient. Trying to get thoughtful and intelligent care at home or in the clinic is as much of a nightmare as being in pain all the time!"

"I'm here. You can count on me."

Melissa says, tears welling up again, "You're a mensch, John. I—well, you know how I feel." She hangs up, laughing and crying at once.

Sometime later, Melissa becomes aware that she is dreaming and seems to awaken. She is standing in Bartlett Gym. She and John are the only ones in the room. It is dark out. Perhaps they forgot to leave at closing time. They move toward each other and begin a slow *pas de deux* of mutual regard during which they spiral closer and closer to each other. She feels growing delight and anticipation. When they are almost touching, she reaches out to him, but they begin to spiral outward again. As they move apart, her delight diminishes. Her clothing seems to be stuck in a bundle. She struggles with it but can't move. In a moment, she is awake and knows that she is on the sofa. As she drifts off again, she wonders if he sometimes dreams of her.

The following night John goes to the library of the Policlinico Le Scotte outside the city's walls, where he is frustrated by his poor command of Italian, and by the limited information that he is able to find in its books and medical databases. Part of him knows that the information he would like to find is unavailable.

He has heard of cases like Melissa's. He is aware that the CDC has had to respond to them, and that they have come up with a case definition. It is not as vague as Melissa's universally positive history. Who could count such cases? This is the stuff for clinical investigation, not health statistics or statistical modeling that amounts either to social "proof" of the obvious or to lies, damn lies and statistics. Even he, who has become a Jack of many trades and a master of none, knows better. Common sense is uncommon, as his professors used to say, and he is pretty sure that he will be able to rediscover his and to dust it off.

Over the next month, she calls at all hours, and he listens and asks questions. She appears to experience a daily peripheral neuritis, with exquisite pain in the lower legs in the afternoon, along with worsened brain fog, papular rash, and general malaise. She then rests like a patient with multiple sclerosis, and sometimes is so sensitive to any and all stimuli that her only relief comes from sequestering herself with tea and a distracting and uplifting film. One day, she fell to her right, especially when she closed her eyes, due to cerebellar symptoms and also had the pill-rolling tremor of Parkinson's disease as well as her usual glass tremor. She often can't find words, substitutes a wrong word without realizing it, or loses her ability to follow a train of thought. She finds it easier to recall memories that are linked to emotion, but cannot speak of them if the emotion is overwhelming.

John can barely stand to think about her suffering—and what's worse, he can feel it when she is telling him about it or when he recalls feeling it. At first this unnerves him, but then he realizes that it is useful: he can empathize with her so fully that he is able to observe her experience from the inside out.

He does not feel desire then. He does feel it when he calls her and debriefs her with respect to her observations. Then their conversations transport him back to the days when they were in love and didn't know it—when their shared contemplation in Harper Library, and their close physical proximity, and the spark of passion ignited by music and warmed by fond familiarity blossomed into an intense union fed by love that was productive of intellectual and erotic ecstasy.

As their union comes to life again, they feed it with their passion to discover the cause of her ailments. He tries not to think beyond that, but he cannot help but see himself rescuing her from Dan. He tries to weaken this vision by taking an interest in the women he sees on the street and in the lab. They take care with their appearance; Italian women scientists seem to him to be the most stylish on the planet. But he cannot read their signals, and they seem ill at ease with him. He feels a certain familiarity that may be respect. One of the women has features that have given rise in his mind to an image of the Mona Lisa coming to life, reaching out of the painting and slapping him for getting fresh. That image is amusing, at least in part, unlike the ones of Laurel with Leon that make him sick with regret when he is unable to block them out. Then the darkness of the life he has created engulfs him. Then he calls Missy and returns to his true self and to their purpose of giving birth to a brainchild that would cure her. He does not go so far as to let himself feel the joy of embracing her—to feel it and lose it again would crush him—or to feel the relief of leaving his failed marriage to make one of meaning and purpose with the love of his life.

One of the great gifts that the city of brick towers has given him—other than Italian lessons at the Dante Alighieri School—is the opportunity to play jazz. Every day he takes a late, two-hour Italian lunch and plays his sax or mouth harp or sings. He has even bought a toy electronic keyboard that he can use to play simple chords to accompany his singing and to write songs.

Every Tuesday and Thursday he takes his instruments through the twilight hour past truck exhaust and brick exteriors to dine free at a boutique hotel restaurant, and then play jazz in its subterranean bar for tips. It takes him back to the days of hope and character formation, and burns off the cancerous growth of hard-won importance that has enslaved him. He dreams of turning his sabbatical into a new beginning. The jazz scene in Siena is wide open. He could make a living playing bebop, blues—even the hot jazz and cool riffs on marching band music that tickle the locals. He may stay for a while and work in one of the old basements repurposed as clubs. He may ask Melissa to come and spend some time with him while they figure out what to do.

And so it is that one night as he is wailing away on his sax in the low-lit smoke-filled room, trying out new riffs that have been forming in his mind, he thinks back on their years together on the south side of Chicago, and plays his way into a memory of the time when they moved into the apartment around the corner from Beaulieu's. She was having a hard time, then. She kept losing her keys. Her grades dipped, too, and she thought that she might not be bright enough to practice medicine. She even talked with Zeke about doing electives in fine art, as he had done. John even remembers the smell in the apartment, which had been saturated with roach spray.

For many minutes he is unaware of thought as the pieces come together into a pattern that he knows is her diagnosis. The aha moment seems to go in slow motion as he expresses her malady as a series of riffs, and then winds up his number and then his set. The audience reaction reveals his amazement, and theirs, which comes from his entanglement with Melissa, their brainchild, and from the intense ecstasy of discovery. The owner signs him for a regular weekend gig with pay.

John seems to float up the street in a daze, barely aware of having gathered his gear. He skims over the cobblestones of a covered street and out to the piazza where families are circling and young people are eyeing each other. He sits at a café table and lets the realization take over his mind and body. He has already questioned her about everything in the way of an expert clinician researcher who has gone back to square one. She does not use household, yard, or institutional chemicals. She never touches the medications she prescribes; those are administered by nurses. She filters her drinking water. She uses old-fashioned bar soap and bar shampoo. And yet she is suffering from chronic recurrent poisoning, which means she and other patients with emerging diseases are ingesting neurotoxins with every meal. They seem to be chronically ill, when in fact they are chronically exposed. Tracing the problem to its source means that the food supply and—by extension—the soil and surrounding habitats and the whole of the biome is poisonous because of human folly. He is shaking. He is flabbergasted

As John absently orders and drinks a glass of local red wine, and then a grappa, he thinks through the causal web and diagnoses it from the source—with question marks for occupational and environmental exposures due to production or use of chemicals, and for alternative routes of exposure such as inhalation and dermal uptake. He does not know enough about the agricultural or chemical industries to make educated guesses about the expected duration or consequences of the problem, or enough about liver enzymes to hazard a guess as to how to group people who might show similar symptoms in relation to which chemicals.

He realizes that he is writing on a linen napkin and that he will have to keep it and see if he has enough Italian to explain that he wants to keep it and pay for it. He calls the waiter, who has come to know him. The waiter shrugs, brings him a fresh one, and waves a hand to signal not to worry. John wonders if he has become well enough known to merit some extra tolerance, or perhaps his tips have won it. He puts a hand over his heart to signal thanks and wonders whether Italians spray their grapes and whether distillation removes any chemicals that are sprayed on crops.

For a time, he lets his mind wander along the ramifications of the causal web. Then abruptly, the backs of his calves creep with the realization that one chemical may have many health impacts, and that a whole cocktail of the kinds of chemicals that end up in food might have many more. As the plaza begins to empty, and he sees the individual instances of his species disperse, and thinks of how each and all are affected by alcohol and tobacco, he realizes that all of the ailments that are increasing—from autism to neurodegenerative diseases to cancer—may be related to chronic poisoning in everyday life. Obesity may be in the causal chains—caused by poisoning and waiting to show its worst outcomes.

He seems to recall that alcohol and smoke contain hundreds of potential carcinogens, and that people metabolize them in varying ways and develop a spectrum of diseases. He thinks of the chimney sweeps who got testicular cancer, and the girls who painted radium on clock faces and got jaw cancer. Each and every one of the chemicals that causes one or more of the occupational illnesses could cause mischief through the ambient environment, and the chemical impact could go undetected indefinitely—even in a clinic or laboratory—until it would be too late to rescue life on earth.

John cannot hold this dark realization for long, or alone. His thoughts turn toward this strange serendipity: in helping Missy he has a chance to help himself—and his patients, his species, and life on earth. But who will believe him? There is no money or status in doing the right thing. There is crucifixion.

The waiter brings him a second grappa on the house. John nods and realizes that his mouth is hanging open and that he must look like he feels, which is as if he has just been told that he does not have long to live. He looks at his napkin drawings and recognizes that there are far too many unknowns for him to come up with a guess as to how small or large this discovery might truly be. He tells himself that so far it is only an idea and only based on one case. He resists the intense urge to share his hypothesis, which he could so easily do.

He knows that the burden of proof lies on those who question convention rather than on those with concerns or truths to share. Proofs are filtered by psychosocial factors that trace back to money and status. Of this he is acutely aware. He knows what he must do to help Melissa and others like her, and it may cost him his status. He has no choice. The staus quo is unacceptable. Some time later, he gathers his gear and wanders across the deserted piazza into the dark night.

Eighteen months later, Melissa is lying down on the floor of the Goddess room at the Nederland ashram, eyes closed. She has been eating hypoallergenic, organic, or better food for over a year, has reduced the fat tissue where poisons are stored, and has become pain-free. She recently did an experiment: she took one-quarter cup of conventional corn oil and recorded the results. She documented the neurotoxicity and then took to her bed for a week, hoping to recover fully in a month or a few. Two weeks into this self-sacrificing setback, Sarah came out to Denver to take Missy to the mountains to recuperate with safe diet, liquids, rest, exercise, and contemplation.

Sarah goes to sit beside her friend and says in a low, tender voice, "I went to the kitchen as you asked and you're right. They use potatoes and tomatoes in almost everything, and no one seems to know the source. And the dairy is pooled and the wheat comes in a big sack from who knows where—whole grain, of course."

"No surprise there. It's hard to pursue my New Kosher diet— all clean food to share with all."

"Would Dan bring up some food from the Boulder Farmer's Market?"

"No."

Sarah releases a sigh and bows her head. "Are you sure you want to stay with him? You could come back to the farm with me…"

"Dan's doing the best he can. I don't remember if I told you this, but his father abused his wife and children. He even used rubber hoses to keep bruises from showing."

"Oh my God! How awful. No wonder he's so shut down. That could help you forgive him."

"It would be easy except that he's never wrong, never has an occasion to apologize, never shows remorse."

"Do you?"

"Too much. I'm my own whipping girl, and he's only too happy to help."

"That's dark."

"That's dualism. You don't feel victimized without victimizing others. Neither pole can persist without the other. Which means every time we take it out on me we create a pattern that tends to perpetuate itself."

"Why don't you come visit me for a month? Just for respite. My sister's family farm is free of added chemicals."

"Tempting. I would love to. But I don't do well when I travel. I may be able to stay with a friend in Boulder. She understands Jewish practice and ... might be able to work with me on embodying the tree of life as a means of creating new frames and constructs for medicine—like Maimonides did in his time."

Sarah says impulsively, "Let's get you in the car and go to Boulder. You can treat us to gas, food, and lodging."

"I can do that, at least." Melissa's brave face falls. She grasps Sarah's hand and asks with an undertone of anxious desperation, "Stay with me?"

"Until you send me home. Actually ... when you're better I'm going to see if I can work here for a while. What you and John have found—plus what you've told Doug and me about habitat destruction—is too important to ignore. I want to do something about it too. I want to be part of what you and John do."

"John's working at a low income clinic in Chicago."

"Really?"

"He lives in his den and talks with me. He's having problems with John Junior. I'm lucky Dan is attentive to our boys."

"Well, at least he's supporting your process, and Dan hasn't left you, and Doug and I are here for you."

"And Pea. She's been wonderful, too."

"Good. The more the better. Are you ready to get up?"

Melissa nods but doesn't move.

"Shall I pack the bags and put them in the car?"

"Would you?"

"Wait here. I'll bring a snack. It's too early for you to try and lose fat and increase your exercise at the same time."

"You're getting to be an expert! Thanks. I … don't know what I'd do without you."

They go out into the crisp air together. The gravel beneath their feet scatters over the dark railroad ties. Around them subalpine firs stretch staunch branches into the thin air, and soften rocky crags. Sarah, who is not yet acclimatized to the altitude, finds her body struggling for air. She does not miss Cayuga because she knows that it will still be there waiting for her when she returns; and she is keen to re-immerse her body in the Rocky Mountains, and to dive deep into the philosophy that Missy is developing. Nothing is more urgent or meaningful than moving humans from the center of their Universe to the periphery of the body of life. This persists in scraps of earth that are as yet healthy despite the careless, radical experiment of modernity, and may yet be rescued by humanity. She is glad to be far from the city, and sorry that Missy and she are alone.

If only John and Doug—at the least—were here!

Sarah helps Missy into the passenger seat of her battered old off-road vehicle, loads the back, and heads down the rutted gravel driveway to the highway down below. They begin the dialogue that Sarah has been gently introducing since her arrival last week, but Missy is losing words and substituting others, and soon stops making sense. As they drive along the ridge, catching glimpses of distant peaks through gaps in the forest, Sarah misses the turn to Boulder canyon. Missy points straight ahead toward another route that appears scenic and uplifting as well as soothing. Their conversation comes and goes in snatches. After half an hour or so, Sarah feels Missy slump down in her seat and glances over to see her crying and putting the seat back.

"Are you okay?"

"It's hitting me now. I should have had a snack. It's just so … hard … it's been hard … I do all this and still … "

Sarah rounds the bend. Ahead is a broken row of relay towers. There is no shoulder on the road, so Sarah turns uphill at the earliest opportunity, does a U-turn, and comes to rest on the shoulder facing downhill.

"Missy?" she says in a soothing tone, "how do you feel now?"

"Not good. I could try my inhaler. Denver pollution has given me asthma—or aggravated it. I could go back on the anti-depressant too. I feel so hopeless."

"I'm going to try something."

"What?"

"I'll tell you in a minute."

"Okay," Missy says hopelessly.

Sarah doesn't know the area well, but is aware that the road will soon slip below a ridge and that she will be able to take a spur road downhill into a stand of evergreens. She does this, and then comes to a stop, turns off all of their electronic devices, and hands Missy out of the car to give her a full-body hug.

Melissa inhales deeply, smiles, and says, "You always make me feel better. You've been radiating health since you became a yoga teacher!"

"Missy, the radio tower and microwave towers had a terrible effect on you. Doug's been telling me how he thinks working in IT is going to give him cancer. What if he's right that it's a hazard—and is impacting you?"

"Radio waves? Microwaves? That's what crazy people say! That's woo-woo!" Melissa laughs darkly.

"What if it isn't? Most doctors you talk to scoff at—or ignore—what you and John have learned. What if they're wrong about this?"

"But how? The radiation is non-ionizing. It's ionizing radiation that damages people."

"Then why do they shield microwave ovens?"

"To keep from cooking people. Are you saying those towers were cooking me? That doesn't make sense. I can still get better when I get away from the poisons."

"I don't know. All I know is that it happened. Why don't we ask John?"

"Yes. Let's. I can't even imagine his coming up with another new diagnosis in such short order, but I can't deny the fact that I feel better already and have no other explanation except you!"

"What diagnosis? Isn't it part of chronic ambient poisoning—the one you guys have been talking about?"

Melissa is silent for a while, and then says, "Radiation poisoning from non-ionizing radiation?"

"I guess so."

"I'm so glad you don't think I'm crazy."

"I've watched things make you sick and seen you remove them and get well. How do doctors miss it?"

"The same way I do."

"Doug's not crazy and neither are you! Our species is turning our Eden into a hell!"

Missy looks around. "The trees… do you think they're shielding us? And the rock up there, they may both block the radiation or radiate life energy just like you."

"I don't know."

"It fits with John's model of my exposure as a more complicated cocktail than he thought, and I may have reached—and gone over—my maximum lifetime dose. My tolerance mechanisms may never recover."

"Or they may." Sarah plops down on the ground, cross-legged, and puts her forehead on her palms. "I wish this was just a theory and not your life."

"At least we have a theory and it has traction." Missy sits down and puts her arm around Sarah's shoulder. "And you—and it—are keeping me alive. And sane."

"And turning you into a doctor for our time."

7

Consequences

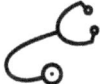

John waits in the doctor's room until the clinic is closed and the others have gone home. It is only seven p.m., which means that it is ten p.m. in New York and a good time to reach Alan at home in Park Slope. John dials and paces nervously as he waits for Alan to answer.

"Alan? Hi. Look, sorry to call so late to ask a favor, but I need to find the best divorce lawyer I can get. I want custody, and it may not be easy because Melissa and I—"

"So what happened already?"

"It's a very long story." His voice is shaking. John clears his throat. "I'll tell you when I come out. I won't need more than a breakfast meeting if—"

"You can stay in the guest room, like last time. Come Saturday evening. I need you to listen to Rachel's playing. She's very talented, plays clarinet, flute, oboe, everything. Piano, cello. We sent her to Music and Art, that public magnet school—the Fame school. It's free, but Debbie's unhappy with it, and what do I know? All I can do is sue them and this is not what she wants. She wants an expensive private school. So what else is new? I need your opinion if Rachel can make it as a soloist, or if she should go into medicine, like I want. Well, it's her life, as long as she doesn't want to be a lawyer. It's a terrible way to live. I've had it.

But who can tell another human being how they should live?"

A parent has to tell a child until she's independent. But when is that? "Al, you're a life saver. I can't tell you how much—but I don't want to impose on Debbie on Shabbos—"

"Debbie likes you, you know that. And she never liked Laurel. She'll want that I should help you get rid of that woman."

John feels the bite of guilt, and an urge to laugh. Alan is sounding more and more like his dead father. John clears his throat and manages to blurt, "I wouldn't ask, but it's been—well—Junior's turned into Thomas. That's how bad it is."

"Where is he now?"

"He's with Doug."

"Is that a good idea?"

"Doug has a better shot at understanding him than I do."

"That we should live to see this," Alan sighs. "Well, take two aspirin and call me in the morning. Better yet, call me from the airport. I'll come pick you up, or you can take a cab. Whatever you want."

"I'll bring my sax. And my harp."

"John, one thing I should tell you right now. Don't answer any questions I don't ask. In case I represent you."

"I'll follow your lead. Melissa said not to trust a lawyer, but I know you'll put my son's wellbeing ahead of everything else."

"How much do you make now?"

John tells him.

"I can tell you right now, you can't afford drug rehab and a divorce too. You can't afford me, and I'm not the best. People will take your money, of course, but you won't get anything for it, that's all I'm saying. But come out for a visit and we'll barter, musical advice for legal advice. If it goes any farther you'll have to barter medical advice."

"Thanks, Al. Any news of April?"

"She's talking to me again. Still a born-again Christian, every few years a different flavor. She's still upset about being put away in the hospital. Post traumatic stress, she's calling it."

"At least she's alive to be upset."

"We don't know if she would be worse off if we did something different."

"True. We never know the road not taken. Listen, Alan, thanks. I can't tell you how much—"

"You can tell me when you come. We're old enough friends we should act like family. Good. So come make a little sunshine with my Rachel. Okay, see you." The line goes dead.

Doug is sitting on his boat, which is rocking in low, foam-touched waves. The rays of the sun are scattering in all directions. He adjusts his visor, switches his cigar to the other side of his mouth, and readjusts his balls for the umpteenth time. The fishing lines are slack. The Kid—Doug can't bear to think of him belonging to John, and so doesn't call him John or Junior—is getting impatient.

"Where are the fish?"

"They aren't biting Kid, they aren't biting."

"We must be doing something wrong."

Doug smiles inwardly. Junior is fishing for a trophy, but Doug is angling for the Kid's sparks. The only one Doug has snagged since John left for New York is the Kid's desire to land a big one. When Doug stopped at the office on their arrival in San Fran, the Kid zeroed in on a framed photo of Doug standing at the end of a dock with his arm around a tuna taller than his head. The Kid wants a picture like that. He wants to see himself beaming beside a sea monster, preferably a swordfish for dramatic effect. He wants to take it home and show it off to his friends. Doug hasn't let slip that Junior may never see those friends again.

Doug knows the tuna are gone and that they will be lucky to find a California halibut, especially as this is the first time he has tried to be his own guide. He knows the hot spots and best times of day but doesn't know how the weather and tides and small fry affect the habits of the fish. "We could troll."

"What's that?"

"That's a way to attract fish by moving so the bait and lure catch the light."

"How do you do that?"

"Move forward slowly."

"You mean reel in the line?"

"There are other ways. Think about it, Kid. Think of a strategy." Doug is constantly amazed by the Kid's situational slowness. The Kid apparently took a top-notch A.P. biology class that's already given him a head start on college, but has been amazed to find that the sea spray tastes salty, that fishhooks have barbs, and that piloting a boat is different from driving a car. He is unable to find the top of a map, describe a lure, or tell one baitfish from another. Doug has to start from square one every time.

Doug thinks fondly of collecting stamps, coins, and bugs, and whittling, and playing with chemistry sets and model railroads—of all the hobbies that engaged him and his friends when they were small. Collecting challenged them to mull things over, to argue, and to assemble, organize, and track a systematized set of objects. Hobbies helped them to hone a whole host of skills. Junior must have missed all that. He can't break down a practical task, carry it out on his own, or troubleshoot it, and shows no signs of manual ingenuity.

The Kid can concentrate, even without pills, but his withdrawal from computer games is an ugly sight. Doug could respect the Kid if he had any inkling of the software or hardware behind consumer electronics, or any perspective on the economics of collusion between marketers and consumerist parents, but the Kid has a dazzling capacity to leap into a plastic box designed to program his mind without worrying whether it will control him completely.

A hundred years ago, the Kid would have been a sucker. Now he is a safety hazard. The Kid's lack of street smarts plus his desperation for button pushing have led him to develop a reckless obsession with the marine radio. Doug explained what could happen if the Kid made crank calls to the Coast Guard, but that only increased his monomania. A few minutes ago Doug found the Kid fiddling with it again. Doug banned it, and backed up his ban with threats, but the Kid doesn't seem to get anything but the war-as-entertainment fantasy games that have overwritten his inborn code.

"We can move the boat forward slowly with the automatic pilot. I'll start the motor."

"This little boat has automatic pilot?"

The Kid is trying to yank Doug's chain again, but Doug doesn't want a bigger boat. He wants this boat. If the Kid understood anything besides *more, more, more!* Doug would have to watch his back every minute. "Kid, this boat has everything I need."

Doug doesn't want to leave the Kid alone, but can't start the motor and watch the tackle at the same time, and so will have to delegate one of those tasks to the Kid. Doug chews his cigar and eyes the bluffs that rise from the beach several hundred yards off the starboard bow. *Wouldn't want to run aground. Better to let the Kid watch the lines than to let him set a course.* Doug takes the calculated risk of leaving the lines to turn the boat seaward into the low chop.

When Doug has strapped himself back in his chair, and they are rocking slowly into quiet, Doug notices the Kid looking above the radar unit. Doug follows the sightline to a trio of seagulls riding the boat's lift. Doug takes heart. Here, away from media and school and drugs, the Kid may be starting to notice the world beyond his joystick coordination.

"Why don't you have kids?" the boy asks.

"It would be too hard on the dogs, Kid. It would be too hard on the dogs. So, Kid, do you miss your friends?"

"High school sucks."

"Miss your family?"

"My family sucks."

"You know Kid, in every family, and in every school, there are people who do just fine in spite of everything. The fact that you're not one of them says a lot about you."

"Don't think you can make me be on their side!"

"Kid, I'm absolutely on your Dad's side, and I'm on yours for his sake, and nobody else in your life means anything to me."

Doug feels like a captain who took along a parrot instead of a passenger. He wishes for the umpteenth time that his dogs weren't afraid of water, and that the Kid had at least one of John's talents. Doug has been looking for signs of the three M's: math, medicine, or music, but the Kid can't even get a note out of a harmonica.

When the Kid has brooded for a good twenty minutes he

brings out the loaded questions. "So, are you married?"

"Guilty as charged."

"How come I didn't meet your wife?"

Doug remembers that John doesn't want Doug to swear or to talk about drugs or sex. He isn't sure where the boundaries are. He suspects that he should take the role of the Uncle who can say things John can't, but Doug chooses his words carefully. "Christy doesn't go out much."

Doug doesn't want to make it too easy, but he doesn't want to discourage the Kid either. The Kid has shown the potential to be canny about people—he has already figured out that Doug is competitive and likes to be praised for his cooking. This unformed ability is one of the few promising signs Doug can find in the Kid. In Doug's world, reading people and touching their likes and dislikes is a crucial art. He keeps mum in a bid to let the Kid sharpen his skills.

Sometime later, when Doug sees buttercream clouds rise above the horizon to the west, he arranges the tackle in resting position and takes the helm. He sets course for the Golden Gate Bridge, which heaves up to the north and east like a toothpick model. When the Kid comes to sit beside him, Doug takes the motor up to full speed.

As they race through the shipping lanes that pass under the grand arch of the Bridge, the Kid shouts, "I didn't know Dad had friends."

Doug notes the intensity in the Kid's voice. The last time he checked, the Kid was enjoying the speed but now his face is pensive. Doug senses that the time has come to speak up for John. When Doug has taken them north out of the shipping lanes, he cuts the speed until the motor is quiet enough to allow conversation. "I hate to break it to you Kid, but every fish we've eaten was more aware of its milieu than you are at this point in your life."

The Kid snorts, but after a pause, says, "I thought maybe you were a—a perv."

Doug laughs, more harshly than intended. "Kid, you're about as attractive to me as a black bear with bald spots that ate too many beans."

"Then why are we staying at a hotel?"

"First, I can keep a better eye on you, and second, I'm not welcome at home just now."

"Why not? Is it because of that Sarah woman?"

Doug wonders how much the Kid heard. Doug knows John doesn't want him to answer this question, but Doug also knows that to be of any real use to the Kid he will have to let loose and ride the currents of their mingled thoughts. Doug holds up his finger for the Kid to wait, cuts the motor to trolling speed, and then motions for the Kid to follow him sternward. When they are strapped into their seats again he says, "Sarah's an old friend of your Dad and Melissa."

"Is that why Dad—is he trying to be like you are with women?"

Doug doesn't try to hide his incredulity. He looks at the Kid until they have full eye contact, fish and lines be damned. "Kid, marriage is a minefield with a million ways to make a wrong move. Your dad made one, and I made a different one."

Even as Doug says this, he doubts it. Maybe they both crushed their wives like bugs. Christy is a butterfly whose wings he pinched too roughly. Laurel is a daddy long legs spider that scuttles under the sink and hides when chased with a broom.

"What wrong move did you make?"

Doug remembers that the Kid is watching him as keenly as Doug is watching the Kid. "I invested some of her money without asking, and lost all of it."

"She's mad over money? Why? You must still have plenty or we wouldn't be on this boat."

"It wasn't the money, it was the principle of the thing. I shouldn't have been so high-handed."

"It's high-handed to see that Sarah woman, isn't it?"

Doug gives the Kid a piercing look with one eyebrow up and one eyebrow down in a frown. "Your dad doesn't want me to talk about Sarah, so I'm just going to say I'm addicted to Sarah the way some people are addicted to drugs, or food, or work, or money. Or computer games."

The Kid doesn't bother to hide his look of triumph. Kid one, Doug zero. "So what mistake did my dad make?"

"Your dad had a soul mate back in college and made the mistake of leaving her. He built up a big dam of denial about it and finally the dam broke and now he's just trying not to drown."

"Mom didn't do anything bad!"

"I'm not going to bad-mouth your mom, Kid, but it always takes two. Always. And your mom is no exception."

As they approach Sausalito, where the sun is shining on calm waters, the Kid asks plaintively, "So is that other woman beautiful?"

"Who, Melissa? No! She's no looker."

"Is she sexy?"

"Not. At. All."

The Kid is bargaining with fate. He asks hopefully, "Is that why he married Mom instead?"

"He left Melissa years before he met your mom."

"He must have left her for a reason."

"Kid, you can only have one top priority in life. One. Your dad's was his career. He left Melissa for his career, but I don't think he'd do it again."

The Kid starts to simmer. After a few minutes he says angrily, "So is my dad having one of those stupid midlife crises where guys act like babies?"

"It's not that simple, Kid."

"Ye-ah-ah. He married Mom and had us. It's his job to take care of us."

"And it's your job to appreciate what you have and work hard and not act like a spoilt brat or endanger your whole family by dealing."

Doug can see that he has overdone it. The Kid's shoulders are up to his ears and his face is set in a scowl. His feelings are hurt. He has no perspective, no rudder, and no way to see that Doug is trying to get the Kid to look into the mirror of his soul out here on the water, where he is safe. It occurs to Doug that the Kid may feel unsafe because he has no safe place inside.

"Look, Kid, you will never meet anyone as smart as your dad. Don't even try to compete with him in that way. Discover your own destiny. Or, if you want to follow in his footsteps, be glad he was there to break trail for you. And be proud of the way he made the most of his talents to help others. He's the best man I've ever known, and he may be the best man you'll ever meet."

The Kid glances at Doug suspiciously and then looks away in a determined sulk.

"The mistake he makes is he gets so intent on doing the best he can at work that he never says no. He sets no limits whatsoever on his profession. So he doesn't protect his core. I work hard and well, but no one micro-manages me. I wouldn't put up with it. Your dad doesn't look after himself that way. If it's any consolation, Kid, he does a better job of looking out for you than he does looking out for himself."

"Gah!"

"The other thing that's different about your dad is he met someone who was perfect for him. Other people get starry-eyed and think they have true love but they don't. He had the perfect mate, but he let his peers and mentors make his choices for him and he lost her. And he made the same mistake with your mom and you."

"She couldn't have been that great if he left her."

Doug feels like a man who is trying to teach a dog to answer the phone. "Don't underestimate her, Kid. She's smart, steadfast, brave, passionate and unique without being weird. And she is perfect for your dad. She loves him like no one will ever love you or me."

"She's not as good as Mom."

"It's not a competition, Kid. Melissa and your dad met when they were young and no one else will ever know them the way they know each other. And, you, Kid, should know your dad may let her go again on account of you, and you had damn well better appreciate it and work to deserve it. If it was me, I'd lose the vengeful wife, and stow you in a clinic and run off. I'd have some fun for the first time in forever and let all the deadbeats on my back deal with their own crap."

The Kid opens his mouth to retort, and then it happens. His yellow line goes taut and the reel starts to spin. Doug can tell by the speed and arc of the line that the lure snagged a big one, and that this beast won't tire for a long time. The Kid starts thrashing.

Doug takes a second to feel the thrill. Chitchat, dialogue and life plummet to the bottom of his priority list. He hears everything at once now, the put-put trolling of the motor, the flapping of a distant spinnaker, the traffic on the Marin side of the Golden Gate, and the slapping of the water on the fiberglass stern. He sees the course of the boat and the direction of the wind and knows he has to cut the motor. Doug sets the Kid's feet back in place and helps him play the line out. Then Doug darts up to cut the motor and dashes back to guide the catch.

Now they are two men alone with a hot reel, the older teaching the younger. Doug's dad never fished, so Doug had to buy that experience for himself, and now he is jazzed to be in a position to pass it on to the son of an old friend. He feels an odd mix of tender protectiveness and raw aggression that must be the paternal instinct he chose never to express. He sees with new eyes what is at stake in John's life, and, at the same time, feels as if he were young again with his old friend.

Doug resolves to do what he can to keep this Kid off the ash heap of life. As the Kid struggles awkwardly with the tension on the line, Doug watches carefully. On the outside, the Kid is like John before he found his physical strength. On the inside, he is not like John the young scholar, who delved into cloisters filled with books, and went out into the wilderness to fill his heart. He is like John the compromised careerist who became a tenacious control freak.

Yesterday, when he gave the Kid a balled up tangle of fishing line they should have thrown away, the Kid spent hours untangling it. Now he wants to force the fish into the boat instead of observing the animal, learning from it, and honoring it. Doug sees potential in raw tenacity, but is not sure how to teach the Kid to apply it judiciously and flexibly. Doug would like to show the Kid how to become the kind of man who is wise enough to choose worthy aspirations, strong enough to achieve them, and powerful enough to lead others to do the same.

Doug takes time to tell the Kid about the fish, its strength, its strategy, and its ways. There is plenty of time for Doug to transmit his limited wisdom on the topic, and his words help the Kid stay focused. After half an hour of struggle, the line goes slack so long Doug thinks the beast is gone, but finally it pulls out the line again, and the Kid plays it out and resumes the physical and mental struggle of wresting the fish from the water. Doug guides the Kid through everything until the silvery tail is hooking back and forth under the clear water near the boat, and the Kid is scooping the net awkwardly around it. The Kid doesn't have the skill to get the fish into the boat. Doug isn't good with the gaff, so he nets the beast and heaves it up.

It is a California halibut, a forty-pound flounder that lands heavily on the deck and stares up at them with side-by-side eyes. Doug could snap freeze it, but he wants the Kid to learn everything the old-fashioned way, so he puts the fish on ice. When they get back to the dock, the Kid will be able to try the filleting knife on solid ground, away from the waves.

The Kid looks disappointed. This fish is not bigger than he is. But when Doug talks it up, which is easy because it is a beauty, the Kid brightens and quickly agrees that he has bagged a great fish and a great story. When the fish is secure, and they have celebrated with a soda, and have talked the story through, Doug scans the horizon. The clouds are still far away. "Let's head south toward the dock, try for another on the way."

"Okay." The Kid adds in a tone that is at once confidential, sympathetic, and gloating, "Maybe you can get one, too."

Doug smiles broadly. "I'd love it, Kid. I'd love it."

After they refuel in Sausalito, and pass under the Bay Bridge, Doug cuts the motor at what he hopes is a promising spot near Alameda. He lets the boat drift in the brisk breeze and settles with Junior into the contemplative quiet of waiting.

After a while, as a reward for work well done, Doug launches into a fish story, the one about the time when he got a blue tuna off the coast of the Baja. He had gone out with a wild and whacky Mexican guide who took him to the mouth of the Bay and handed him diving gear and a harpoon rig and no instructions. Doug figured out how to use the rebreather and harpoon, and eventually nailed a big tuna. He was about to surface and wave to the guide when he saw a shark approach, apparently drawn by the tuna's blood. The Mexican waited until the last minute before taking Doug in, and laughed all the way back to port.

The Kid loves the story. "Are there sharks here?"

"No kid, no. That was a story to keep the prisoners on Alcatraz."

Doug is enjoying himself now. He is happy to have snared another of the Kid's sparks, and to have discovered that when the Kid listens, he looks just like John did back when they solved math problems at the study table in Regenstein Library. Doug had forgotten how John hunted for solutions, and is glad to see that intensity come back to life.

Doug puts out the lure of another great fishing story and reels the Kid in. Then he stops. He wants to use stories sparingly and so reveal the magic of the rare pleasure. The Kid doesn't know that there is more to life than the demon's lair of plenty. Doug also wants to teach the Kid that there's more to learning than getting A's in school. He has noticed that any little part of the Kid's mind that has not been overwritten by the marketers and designers of video games and rap music has been programmed by schools to get A after A after A. The Kid lives in a Brave New World minus a governing intelligence, a situation that is a problem and also a key to redemption. All Doug has to do is to slip some code into the Kid's program that engages the Kid in getting self-awarded A's in vision and originality. Doug says as casually as he can, "Don't let your schooling get in the way of your education."

"What does that mean?"

"That's Mark Twain for school doesn't teach you how to live your life."

The Kid frowns at him suspiciously.

"You do know who Twain is?"

"Yeah-uuuh. Huckleberry Finn."

"Twain was a great humorist who honed his style working for the San Francisco papers, back when they were the SNL of their time."

The Kid's suspicion deepens. Doug smiles inwardly. The Kid's doubt is unnecessary. Doug is restricting his rough play to sarcasm and satire. Exaggeration and fabrication would only fuel the flames under the hot air balloon of the Kid's mind, and Doug doesn't want the Kid floating up into the ozone on his watch.

"Saturday Night Live is ephemeral, funny when fresh. Twain's been funny for a hundred years."

"What's so funny about saying that schooling gets in the way of schooling?"

"It's wit, Kid, and it's no good if you have to explain it."

The Kid nods sagely. He doesn't want to be the guy who

doesn't get it.

"Since this is the end of the twentieth century, I'll add that you can't learn from memes or messages either. They only get in the way."

"If you know so much, why don't you get along with your wife?"

Doug follows the Kid into deeper waters. "I, uh, she's, uh, delicate. In some ways. And I'm not."

"Why doesn't Dad get along with Mom?"

The Kid sounds truly puzzled, which prompts Doug to reflect on his own troubled union. He muses aloud, "I don't know, Kid. But it's like this, when you get married, you get this gift box marked 'open when the easy happiness runs out.' And when it runs out, and you open that box, you look inside and find the work that comes with the marriage. The hardest work is the deep changes you have to make to get on with your partner. It may be a lot or a little, but it'll be something you didn't choose, and may be the hardest work you'll ever do."

"So people run away from that?"

"When you face the question of whether or not to give up, you have to ask yourself if the work of the marriage is work you should do anyway, either because it's part of your life work, or because you have to do it to get on with people you care for, including yourself. If the answer is yes, you buckle down and do it. If the answer is no, you face the hard question of whether to stay together or not."

"So what's my dad's life purpose?"

"I don't know, Kid, but I'm sure you're part of it."

"You keep saying my dad's smart, but if he's smart why can't he get along with Mom?"

"That's a good question. Nobody who gets married expects it to take work, and if you're already working to the max, like your dad, you may be overwhelmed by it. Besides, it takes more than smarts. It takes character. If you're lacking in certain areas, you try to build them up, and you get all the help you can. That's why your dad is turning to old friends, like me. We're in the self-help capital of the world right now, and your dad is checking it out."

"You mean my dad hasn't got any character?"

"He has an oversupply in some areas. Which you would know if you had tapped into them."

The Kid seems to accept that answer. Doug is pleased. He is so contented that it takes him a few minutes to notice that after the Kid visits the head, and flushes the marine toilet, he doesn't return. When Doug does notice that the Kid is missing, he drops his cigar into the water sloshing at his feet, leaves the tackle, and bounds into the cockpit. The Kid is fiddling with the marine radio. Doug is angry, but he is prepared to put his temper to good use. He takes a giant step over to the Kid and grabs the microphone out of his hand.

The Kid says, "I didn't touch it."

"Kid, if you believe that, you're in bigger trouble than I thought."

"I was just—"

"Did I tell you not to touch that?"

"I was only—"

Doug's gut decides, without formal analysis, that it is time to use his size and strength to express some tough love. Junior is on the brink of destruction and words will not bring him back. Doug knows that the Kid is skinny like John; is a strong swimmer; and, though sixteen, a virgin to physical confrontation.

He hooks his right elbow under the Kid's neck and his left under the Kid's knees, picks up the Kid who thrashes like a big baby —and hauls him up the step to the port side. Doug feels a sudden intense pain in his triceps. The Kid twisted his mouth around and closed his teeth on Doug's arm.

Doug bites the kid's shoulder hard enough that he stops thrashing. When Doug reaches the port gunwale, he heaves the Kid over into the frigid waters of the Bay. When the Kid surfaces, he is thrashing so much he nearly sinks. Doug folds his arms and waits. After a while, the Kid stops thrashing and begins to tread water. He spits out a stream of seawater and shouts angrily, "I'm freezing! I could get sick!"

"You're uncomfortable, Kid. And you have not asked for my assistance."

"Pull me in now!"

Doug cups his hand behind his ear and mimes listening. "Did you ask me something?"

The Kid is beginning to catch on. He treads tensely for a minute and then says with forced calm, "Please pull me in!"

Doug grabs the rope cleat on the gunwale with his right hand and stretches his left out. The Kid grabs it. Doug pulls up until the Kid's waist is at water level. The Kid scrambles to grab the boat, but Doug extends his arm and dangles the Kid. "Repeat after me. I will not touch the radio."

"Come on—"

Doug plunges the Kid into the water and lets go. When the Kid surfaces again, and has grown calm again, Doug cups his hand behind his ear again, and says, "You were saying?"

The Kid glares up at him. "I will not touch the radio."

"Good." Doug reaches out again and pulls the Kid up until

he is dangling crotch high in the water. "Repeat after me, my actions have consequences."

The Kid blows away the water that is running down from his hair over his mouth. "My actions have consequences."

Doug drops the Kid again. When the Kid resurfaces, and calms down again, and is treading water, Doug says, "Repeat after me. I will never bite another living thing."

"I'm glad to hear it."

Doug smiles inwardly. The Kid is feisty. Doug likes it, but will not take the hook. "This ain't a negotiation, Kid. When I tell you to do something, you do it. From now on." Doug cups his hand behind his ear again and says, "You were saying?"

The Kid spits angrily, "I will never bite another living thing again."

Doug reaches down and pulls the Kid up to the gunwale, from which point the Kid scrambles into the boat and lies abjectly in the bottom, shivering. He scrambles to his feet and stands, hugging himself. He is wary but steely, and resolute.

"Go get fresh clothes, Kid." When the kid has gotten dry clothes from his bag, and Doug is watching him change in the cockpit, Doug says, "We're going in. I know what to tell your Dad."

The Kid's face opens in triumphal resentment. "You've been spying on me!"

"I've been planning your education. Which will continue at the dock with you getting a picture and cleaning this fish."

"I'm not gonna—"

"Repeat after me. My actions have consequences."

The Kid is stiff-as-a-board livid, and silent.

"Would you like another swimming lesson? Or do you want

to say it?"

The Kid swallows hard. "My actions have consequences."

"All right, all right. Loosen up, now, have some fun. You got a great fish, and you're about to get a very long break from school."

The Kid opens his mouth to speak, but thinks better of it. As he helps to put away the gear, he tries to sulk, but is too awake from the swim and too excited about the fish. He sits up front with Doug as they head in to port, and starts talking like a prisoner who has measured his guard's power and decided he could meet it. The Kid's stream of consciousness reminds Doug that he, too, was once an ingrate teen ready to pass judgment on the world and everyone in it, and to defy rules without considering any consequences. The Kid is a lot like Doug, which means he may be able to channel the Kid's callow confidence into something constructive.

As they approach the dock where Doug is berthing his boat for the week, he is relieved to see his favorite guide walking out from the shingled shop. One of the Guide's grandchildren, who have explored nooks and crannies of trouble the Kid has yet to discover, must have been on the lookout for their return. As they draw up to the guest moorage, the Guide rubs his five-day growth of grizzled beard, pulls down his fishing hat, and leans his bulging belly over the cleats. Doug tosses him a line and has the Kid hop out to help tie up.

When the boat is secure, and the Kid has shown the Guide the fish, the Guide takes it to the hanging station and shoots some trophy photos of the boy with his arm around it. The Guide takes a few more of the boy holding the fish in his arms like a swooning princess and then sets them up at the cleaning station with a hose and a knife. When he learns that the Kid has never filleted, he pushes up to the Kid's side and grabs his hands.

The Kid looks a little frightened, as if intimidated by the knife, the flesh of the dying fish, and the Guide's big black hands, which are scarred and callused. While Doug holds his breath and stares, the Kid cringes at the touch of the fish's scales and grimaces at its guts. When he splits the fish's belly with surgical precision, the kid's expression settles into shock, as if he is making his first stomach-lurching link between eating a fish and taking its life. At least the Kid is getting his unskilled hands into something other than trouble.

In Doug's day this ritual was an integral part of childhood, even for the city-bred, but he is suddenly and strangely worried that the Kid may lose a finger to the keen-edged knife. He puts all his faith in the Guide, who reminds him of a grandparent easing a wiggly toddler into a snowsuit. Doug is grateful to the Guide. He has been Doug's favorite since he bagged the tuna in the office photo. Doug hires this guide whenever he wants to be sure that a client or a friend catches a big one.

Doug knew about the Guide's grandkids, but only just learned about the Oakland street kids who have become his de facto grandkids, along with the sons of a growing network of dads who have lost faith in themselves, the neighbors, the churches and the system. This network has extended across the Bay Bridge to take in a set of guilty-hearted gay artists who won't touch a fish but will fight for their sons' right to catch one. Doug is part of that network now, and intends to behave as if he is angling for Best Customer Award. He may even pull some wayward teens off the streets and drag them here to meet this wise elder.

Doug knows that the Guide has all the latest fish-finding equipment but suspects he uses it only to comfort technophiles. He seems to locate fish by using his instincts, perhaps the same ones used by birds of prey. He has also set up the dock to contain wayward teens, so that everything they need is at end of the dock where the water is deep, including a grill, ice chest, and some chairs, which means that Doug and the Kid will get to watch the sun set over the Bay while dining on some of the best halibut on the West Coast.

The Kid doesn't notice any of this, but he does notice that he has become one of the guys. He seems happy and even eager to help as they transfer the boat to its slip, say a long goodbye to the Guide, and pack their photo and remaining fish in the car. By the time they make their way to the small hotel north of the Golden Gate Bridge, the Kid is ready for the forgetfulness of sleep.

Doug wishes that were possible. The hardest moment of the day is yet to come. It is time to call John and recommend a curriculum for the Kid, and Doug wants the Kid to hear every word, even though it may cost them both the privilege of several days of pleasant fishing. While the Kid is in the shower, Doug calls John on the bedside phone and learns that Alan is thriving and that Laurel is blaming Junior's problems on John and threatening to take sole custody. John sounds so tired that Doug skips over the chitchat and, as the Kid is coming out of the shower, says, "Okay, Long John, here's the scoop. You've got a great kid, but he has some bad habits, as you know. Yeah, I know, don't we all. But he needs a big change, and he needs it right now."

The Kid is outraged. He puts his pajama bottoms on angrily, standing on the legs so they get stuck below his knees. "I want to talk to my dad!"

"Hold on a minute, John." Doug rotates the mouthpiece above his head to talk to Junior. "From now on Kid, you earn all your privileges."

Doug swings the phone down again. "Melissa thinks you can change a habit in a month, but that's if you want to. He's going to need three. A year would be better."

The Kid pulls up his bottoms and stalks toward Doug. "I want to talk!"

"Hold on a minute, John." Doug reaches his free hand into his pocket and pulls out a set of handcuffs. He swings the phone up again and says calmly to the Kid, "If you don't shut up, sit down, and listen, I will handcuff you to the chair and duct tape your mouth."

"Doug—" begins John.

Doug swings the phone down and stares the Kid in the eyes as he says to John, "His main problem is he's devious. He's also arrogant and ignorant, which makes him a danger to self and others. He isn't addicted to drugs, but he is addicted to consumer electronics, and it is the eleventh hour for instilling strengths before his weaknesses overwhelm him."

The Kid looks down. His face fluctuates between anger, shame, and the chilly realization that Doug sees through him, and so does his dad. Doug has the instinctive feeling, or maybe he is only kidding himself, that the Kid is relieved to be taken in hand. Whatever the reason, he stays quiet for the rest of the call.

"What do you suggest?" asks John tensely.

"It can't be me because I'm backed up at work, or you because you have other business to attend to, but I know a skipper who could take him for a three-month trial period, with a full year if he passes muster. The setting would be ideal because Junior needs to get out into the world and yet be under someone's eye every minute."

"Yachts and drugs tend to go together," John observes.

"The skippers I know come in two flavors, degenerate and incorruptible. This one's the latter. You can put your faith in him. He has problems with women, yeah I know, don't we all, but he's a good role model in other respects."

"How did you get to know him?"

"He was captain on a small cruise Christy and I took a few years ago. He's an incredible leader, and he's putting together a crew for a long Pacific voyage. He doesn't know the owners, but the captain is in charge on the water, and this one's good with all kinds."

"Could Junior get any kind of school credit for it?"

"Let's not worry about that right now."

"Gotcha. It sounds like a much better option than treatment. I'll talk to Laurel about it."

"When you see her tell her the Kid bagged a big halibut. Yeah, a forty pounder, and he skinned it and cooked it, too. No, I'm not kidding. The Kid is capable."

The Kid is somewhat mollified by the acknowledgment of his efforts and success, but when Doug puts down the receiver he says resentfully, "You were spying on me!"

"I was evaluating your character, Kid. The good news is you have some, and can develop it if you get the right curriculum, with some life experience and good hard work. For starters."

The girls are clustered at the near end of the court. The coach tells Tiffany and her teammates to spread out, but they all want to be in the same place at the same time, and as near to the ball as they can get. John can't see Tiffany, who is on the other side of a player several inches taller and many inches wider. When the ball thumps the backboard, and the girls come up the court en masse, John is surprised at how ripe they smell. They are approaching puberty.

John can't believe how mature his daughter is, or how hard she is trying to figure out what to pay attention to. *I don't want to let you down, Tiff.* He gathers his resolve and turns to Laurel, who is sitting beside him on the bleachers. "Can we agree to take Junior out of school for a year at sea?"

Laurel nods, and then shakes her head, eyebrows high. She is pale with anger.

John persists. "It's a big step. We won't see him much. But I think it's for the best."

Laurel has been sitting on a clutch of blame eggs for years, and won't budge before they hatch. She says bitterly, "You've taken everything from me, even Leon."

John is shocked that Laurel would blame him for that fiasco, and even more surprised she is speaking loudly enough that other parents can hear. She used to keep up appearances at all costs. She has lost her perspective, her pride, and her pretense.

"Lucky for us, we've always worked well together. When Junior is back on track we can talk through the rest, do the best with what we have, set a good example for the kids."

"We? You mean you."

John gathers his willpower and says quietly into her ear, "I'm sorry for my part in all this. I should have taken Junior in hand years ago. And Leon wouldn't have entangled you if I had spent more time with you."

"I don't regret Leon."

John's neck tenses. He isn't sure which is more loathsome to him, the thought of touching her, or her romantic notions about

Leon. He shakes it off. "I'm happy in the den, and you're welcome to do as you like, if you're discreet."

"You want to live together and not sleep together?"

"We might change our minds in the future, but—"

"No! I want to quit that part of my job. I've always felt like—" Laurel looks around and lowers her voice, "like I was servicing you."

John senses that this is very painful for her, and realizes he has many apologies to make. "I'm sorry. We never had easy chemistry, and I didn't know how to make up for it."

"You've forgotten it because of her."

Did I forget? John is asking Melissa in his mind. He talks to her all the time now. He is grateful that she is always with him.

I don't know John, what did you feel?

I had sex with her but I don't think I made love to her.

If it's true, and Laurel doesn't know it, it would be cruel for you to bring it up. She thinks you made love to me again, you know.

"I didn't sleep with her," he says aloud to Laurel.

"Why would you think that that matters?"

John has no reply.

"You love her and you sleep with me. I'd have more respect for you if you slept with her. What you do is just—sick. It's cold."

John is about to mention his feelings about Laurel's affair when he notices that she has just given him permission to sleep with Melissa. He blurts eagerly, "You want me to sleep with her?"

Laurel has no reply.

Did sleeping with him make it better?

"Did sleeping with Leon make it better?"

"Yes. Until I found out it had to do with *you*. Now it's—hell."

John feels Melissa's hand resting on his shoulder, steadying him. He takes a deep breath and says calmly, "I'm sorry I didn't see it coming."

That's why they call it blind ambition.

John laughs. *Thank you, Melissa. Thank God for you. I couldn't face this without you.*

"It isn't funny!"

"I'm not laughing at you, or at us. I'm laughing at how blind I was."

Laurel looks at him suspiciously. "You've changed. How can I trust you again?"

"We'll come to a new understanding, when we get through this."

Laurel asks incredulously. "You really love her, don't you?"

"She—" he halts. Love and longing grip his throat. He nods mutely.

"Why couldn't it be me?"

John shakes his head. Denial and excuses disappear. He is face to face with a question for which he has no answer. He wonders if he ever tried to love her the way he loved Melissa, or if he expected to feel it automatically, or if he didn't expect to love her at all.

They do not speak again until after the second quarter of Tiffany's game, when John realizes that he can still sense Laurel's moods. She is softening. He presses his advantage. "I'll stay in my current position until we figure things out. You can count on me."

Laurel shakes her head. She is near tears now. "We've lost everything."

"We haven't lost the children. They'll be all right if we work together. And we have the house."

Laurel's eyes redden. "How can we have people over?"

John suppresses a laugh. *That is the least of our problems, wouldn't you say?*

No. Not to Laurel. Not to your wife. Talk to her.

"Well, no more dinners for my colleagues. They'll never be able to think of anything but Leon. And the relatives will be fixated on Junior's absence."

"Do you want a divorce?"

"Do you?"

"I don't know." Laurel whispers, "If we divorce, Leon wins."

8
Continuation

Melissa and John are standing in a darkened alcove beside the elevator column of Regenstein Library, peering into a humidity-controlled display case holding several browning books, one propped open on a canted stand. Melissa brushes her fingertips over the transparent case and says, "My friend Katherine says that when her mentor studied in Dublin years ago, the Book of Kells sat right out on a podium in the University library. Students could walk right up and touch it. But they didn't. They were in awe of it. And now it's sitting in a clear cage like this one, where fingers and breath can never reach it."

John's breath stirs the hair on her neck as he says in a low voice, "Can we live without touching the things we treasure?"

She turns and puts her palm on his breastbone. In this light his green eyes look almost brown. "Anything is possible."

John puts his hand over hers. Melissa squeezes his hand, withdraws hers slowly and touches her fingers to her lips. She turns back to the case, where she sees Doug and Sarah's faces hovering on the opposite side. Sarah's expression is radiant but hesitant, and Doug's is animated and yet portentous. They seem to be pausing between bouts in their affair. Melissa hopes that they won't go at it, or go home.

"It's a reminder," Sarah says with a significant look at Melissa.

"An artifact can be taken as a symbol of the hidden treasures that are always with us, and can never be sealed off."

Melissa smiles at Sarah and then turns to John distractedly. "Look! It's in Latin! Maybe it's an *Index Medicus*?"

John laughs lightly. The medical reference books they used as students have gone digital, which makes the old volumes as obsolete as this relic. Doug and Sarah exchange glances. They feel as if they are spending time with twins who share a secret language. Even so, they all understand, because of the back channeling that went into organizing this day of reunion, that John and Melissa will be making their decision today.

"Was it that one?" John points to a table near the central staircase.

"You mean our study table?" Doug asks. "Wrong floor."

"Really?" John and Melissa say together. Then they look at each other and say, "Jinx."

"I want to see if the Oriental Institute is open," Sarah says to Doug.

"Perfect," he replies sourly. "We can have a group grope with the mummies."

Sarah grabs Melissa's arm and rushes down the stairs and out of sight. As John and Doug follow slowly after them, John tries not to think of what happened when he went to pick up Doug and Sarah at their room in the Drake Hotel. He arrived a few minutes after the appointed time, and was halfway through the partly open door of their room when he heard a whoosh followed by a thwack. It could only be the sound of a cracking whip. He ducked out, pulled the door shut, and knocked loudly. When it creaked open, he saw Sarah standing with her right hand on the doorknob and her left hand clutching a whip. Her face was red with distress. She was nearly naked. Behind her, Doug was tied to the bed, his face contorted in rage, his erection as tall and stiff and red as the bloom of a bromeliad.

John turned and ran, trying to think of them as patients. Hearing about Doug's problem and seeing it are two different things. John felt a cocktail kick of shame, dread, and, finally, as he ran down the stairs to the mezzanine lobby, sodden sorrow.

Sarah had run after John and said, "I can't leave him like this. If I leave him now, he'll break down and buy this, and then he'll never be free of it."

"Can't you, uh, change it up?"

"I did. And it worked—until now."

"You must care about him to absorb all that—that—violence."

"I must," Sarah replies with a look of disbelief. "We contain it pretty well."

John had put all that out of his mind while Melissa was with them, but now that he is walking down the stairs with Doug, John says, "Sarah caught up with me this morning and we talked a bit, and I mentioned I'd be glad to work with you on your addiction, if you want. Given what happened with Junior and this morning, it's a bit late to worry about overstepping boundaries."

"I'm sorry about the morning. Things got out of hand before—"

"Don't worry about it. We should go fishing on our own and talk about all the tough stuff, how we are with parents and wives and lovers, and how we are in bed."

"And don't forget politics and religion and money."

John laughs. "Should be easy if we're honest about the rest."

"This is what I get for starting you on self-help."

"In medicine, it's all in a day's work."

When the four friends regroup on the front walk, they turn toward the main quadrangle entrance across the street. Melissa dawdles so that she and Sarah can follow, and Melissa will be able to watch John walk, and see the way he moves his head and narrow hips, which she once thought odd but now thinks perfect. *How did I go so long without seeing or touching him?*

As the four enter the unseasonably hot quadrangle, which is crowded with Alumni visiting for Reunion weekend, Melissa keeps up her conversation with Sarah while she watches. "I can't believe you torched your journals on the beach at Jackson Park."

"You liked my ritual, admit it."

"I liked when we wrote bad things on pieces of paper and burned them. But you spent hours and days and years recording our lives in your journals. I wouldn't have burned those."

"I wrote reams about nothing. I would have burned them last winter but something held me back. This time I was ready to let them go."

Sarah lifts her hair over her shoulder. "So is your counselor helping with Dan?"

"We were in a cold place, and now it's warmer. I'm sure we'll always be friends. One way or another." Melissa and Sarah follow the men out of the quadrangle and across the street to the Oriental Institute, where they enter the stone building and stand to the side of the busy interior corridor. Scholars with black leather briefcases are darting up and down the halls and stairs. The four feel like tourists who have taken a wrong turn until they find a series of discrete signs that point them to the basement, and on to the collection currently on display.

Melissa remembers the museum as a grotto dominated by a huge, black stone bull. Now, samples from the early, productive excavations in Egypt and Sudan are arrayed in cases along the walls like fine china in an upscale store. She likes the look of the relics that reveal and conceal ancient mysteries, the displays of symbolic art, and the discrete plaques with cryptic numbers. The gallery reminds her of the artifact-packed museum at Mount Olympus, minus the gorgeous view.

Sarah stops in the middle of the first gallery. She holds up her hands to signal silence, looking like a teacher preparing to wow her class. She pulls a notepad from her tote bag, waves it like a signal hankie, and then rips off four sheets and deals them out. "Okay, before we talk, let's play a game. Each of us will take a piece of paper and write down four words to describe this place. No academic words like archeology or Egyptology. Okay?"

"Are we going to burn them?" Doug asks with a smirk.

A woman in field clothes looks up from a hieroglyphics display, a wry expression on her face.

They each fish out a pen, write something on a tiny sheet, fold it, and put it into Sarah's cupped hands. She flattens and shuffles the papers behind her back. Then she pulls one out and reads, "Death, taxes, collection, expenses."

Doug and John both look at Melissa. Melissa asks, "What are the rules?"

"We guess who wrote them. We all knew that one was yours," Sarah says to Doug, going on to the next paper. "Tomb, death, selfishness, vanity."

Melissa gasps. She whirls on John and accuses, "You decided!"

Sarah looks at Doug, who shrugs. Sarah looks at the paper again, and then at John.

John replies. "The big picture comes first. You taught me that."

"Which one?" Melissa has been dallying outside of time,

drunk on John and her daydreams of living with and loving him. His pessimistic self-negation suggests the end of her sublimity.

John fixes her eyes as if setting a dare. "I'll come to you. If you say the word."

"What's going on?" Sarah asks.

"Melissa guessed who wrote that one," Doug replies, and then says to Melissa, "Well, Miss M, you get two bonus points for that."

John smiles. "Better give her seven. The kick went between the posts."

Melissa says tremulously, "I want eight points for running it into your end zone." Before she can think about what she is doing, and before he has time to wonder what she means, she bounds to him and presses her chest and lips against his.

Doug covers his face with his hands and says between his fingers, "Okay, okay. Eight points for the touchdown and two-point conversion."

Melissa releases John. *Wet lips, no bolt of lightning. I must have imagined the passion. That will make everything easier.* "We should have had sex until the fire went out, followed the old story of desire, abandon, sin, repentance, and confession. And begging forgiveness."

Doug says, "This has to be worse than you seeing us."

"Seeing you what?" Melissa asks.

Sarah replies, "Doug and I were, uh, busy, when John arrived."

Melissa laughs incredulously. "You two get an early start."

John shakes his head but keeps his eyes on Melissa's. He is only just catching up with the kiss.

Melissa's fierceness fades. Gravity is on the verge of pulling her apart. Her eyes appeal to John's. "I hope you brought plenty of spit and glue with you."

John smiles bravely, but his eyes redden at the corners. "I can find some."

Sarah says quickly, "Okay, let's finish the game." She reads the next sheet, "Digging, discovering, looting, hoarding."

Melissa laughs. "Yours, Sarah?"

"You got it. And yours is: tomb, idolatry, spirit, metamorphosis."

Doug says, "Maybe you went to the same school."

Sarah takes a deep breath and looks around. "You know what I like most here? The lighting."

Doug smirks. "That's deep Sarah, really deep."

Melissa says, "No, I get it! Who are museum displays for? If archeologists wanted to honor the dead, they'd leave relics in their resting places. If they wanted to use them for research, they'd warehouse them. This is a way of showing off things that have monetary value because they're rare. Their meaning may always be a mystery, especially to non-archeologists, so they show them off the way stores display exclusive goods!"

Sarah says with a laugh, "Doug was right. I just like the way they lit the exhibit."

"Oh! How embarrassing. Me too, very nice."

John laughs. He loves that Melissa can find meaning in a piece of pita and then go on to savor its taste and take its nourishment. Life is rich around her, high and wide and deep and open, nothing like life around Laurel, which is like pushing a passage into an unexplored cave with his helmet scraping the roof and his arms pinned to his sides. John feels hopeful. He can't believe Melissa kissed him like that, in front of other people. She was always fastidiously private. The kiss was a stunt, like his dare, but he felt in her a tense arousal that is lingering in his body, reminding him of the dreams he has when he is falling asleep a thousand miles away but is transported to her bed, and she turns to him, and they lay together, and he feels the sweet light of release.

When they have left the museum and are walking toward the lake, the sun burns John's scalp through his thinning hair. He doesn't care. While he is walking and talking with Doug about fishing in California, he stays as close to Melissa as he can, and pictures himself moving to Denver with Junior. John wants to reach out and put his hand on Melissa's shoulder, but he knows that timing is everything, and that this is not the time.

Without having discussed it, the four friends turn toward the Midway and go east to Rockefeller chapel. They walk up the front stairs to the pale stone edifice, where Doug asks Melissa, "You going to send your kids here?"

"I hadn't thought of it. If they wanted to, I might not say no."

"You've changed your tune."

"Have I? Well, the classes were good. ... But now you mention it, I'd push for a campus someplace safe and sunny, where they can't take the risks we did."

Melissa stumbles and finds that her heel is on John's toe. She looks up into his intense eyes, which are glinting green in the sun, beckoning her to join him in his skin, now and forever. *I'd be a fool to let him go.* "I'm sorry. This is—confusing!"

John says with a sly, breathless smile, "Confusing or difficult?"

Melissa feels like an ice skater whose right blade is gliding toward the joy of John while her left blade is heading loyally home toward her family. She is about to hit the ice. "Yes!"

"Good. I'd hate to think it was clear, or easy."

Melissa is flustered now. His touch is taking over her mind.

She is like a drunken woman at a bar who knows the last drink was a bad idea but can't resist the next. She wants to grab him, pull him into the chapel, and take him then and there under a pew, visitors be damned. *No! Don't let romance overwhelm reason!* Melissa rushes ahead to grab Doug's arm and pull him toward Blackwood Avenue and the dormitory. She regrets it immediately. Escaping John for Doug is like running from a charismatic movie star into the clutches of his agent, who can pull your strings, and has no scruples.

Doug says, "You know, if you wanted to take responsibility for the consequences of your actions, you'd marry John."

"Consequences to whom?"

"To yourselves. You haven't done the hard work you were born to do together. Imagine the clinic you could create."

"What about 'first do no harm'? It's the first tenet of our shared work."

"What about the harm you're doing each other? Who'll look after you if you two don't?"

"What if we were born to look after each other from a distance?"

"Fucking ingrates." Doug tries to smirk. "Some people would kill for what you've got."

Melissa can see Doug is unhappy, so she resists a retort and tries to be the one who turns tough stuff into jokes. "That's really romantic, Doug. Very appealing."

John is pleased when Melissa falls back to walk with him, and Sarah rushes up to take Doug's arm. It reminds him of their first walk to Beaulieu's. He is so lost in the feel of her that he loses all sense of time, and is surprised to realize when they reach Beaulieu's and take their seats at a table that he barely noticed

Blackwood Dorm.

Sarah says, "This University is no place to learn about the nature of the mind, or to grow in emotional or spiritual literacy. But what mainstream school teaches that?"

"Right! I mean our analytical minds can handle, what, four variables, seven on a good day? And we live in an infinite universe," Melissa says. "Someone on the faculty should have noticed that there was an eentsy gap between our capacity for rational thought and the immensity of what we hope to understand, and that there was no reason to push us so hard when we could accomplish so little in the long run."

John says neutrally, "Discovery requires unusual mental effort early in life."

Missy adds, "It's like any kind of conditioning."

"We pushed each other. We competed instead of cooperating," Sarah says.

Doug says, "Miss M, you missed a lot of education that was going on here. A lot of us experimented with psychedelics, the paranormal, biofeedback, psychoanalysis, Jungian psychology, you name it. People pushed the envelope all the time, in class and out of it."

Melissa counters, "And yet, while students elsewhere were making love not war, and taking action to end sexism and racism and corporatism and poverty, we were doing homework as if we could study our way out of the Cold War, economic imperialism, and perpetual war. We only studied our way out of common sense, not to mention happiness."

John shakes his head. "Think of the times. Bruno Bettelheim left a concentration camp and came here to teach autistic children how to live in the world. And Weitzman went through that hell and made sense of it. Their accomplishments were extraordinary."

"But think of the Manhattan Project and supply side economics. The University is like a big calculator that anyone with money or power can use to punch in a formula and get the answer they want. And damn the consequences. There's no moral center, no higher vision, and no apology for harm done; only ambition, egoism and depression."

Sarah contradicts, "There was a big picture at SSA."

John persists, "We were here at a hard time. Think of slavery, immigration, the stockyards, the Great Depression, World War II, the Korean War, the Vietnam War, the assassinations, and the riots. The area around us had been torched only a few years before we arrived."

Doug says, "What do you expect of the faculty, anyway, omniscience?"

"Insight; perspective; integrity; an ability to synthesize analyses based in divergent paradigms; a view of the big picture. This faculty has no frontal lobes, no limbic system, and no heart at all. It preserves fragments of rationality the way anatomists preserve organs in jars."

"You can't judge the past by the standards of the present," Sarah replies.

"Neuroscience has come a long way," John observes. "And education too."

"You wouldn't be having this conversation at all if you hadn't had the benefit of the ivory tower education you like to complain about," Doug points out.

Melissa shakes her head in frustration. "I still say mindless analysis leads to nihilism."

Sarah says, "You just don't like this place because it took

John away."

"And I'm not sorry," John says. "I'm glad you're here, now, exactly as you are."

"Don't do that." Doug rolls his eyes. "Don't drop me in a vat of syrup."

Melissa is suspended between hope and despair, grateful for the conversation, which is honest and probing and potent, and powerful enough in its purpose to envelop her in the light of loving reason. Before she can say it, though, Sarah speaks.

"Okay, let's play another game. Everyone think of a good memory of our time here and tell it. We'll go around and around the table taking turns until we all stop because someone comes up with one that we all agree is best. Okay?"

"A little loose on the house rules, there, Sar."

"Right. No proper names and no editorial comments."

"What if we don't stop?"

"Then we keep getting happier until lunch arrives."

"Well, if you put it that way, roaches and cockroaches," jokes Doug.

"And no irony or sarcasm. The win is joy."

Doug shrugs with his face and they go counterclockwise around the table, John, Melissa, Sarah and Doug again. "Beaulieu's, Mintel's class, Blackwood Hall, Friday nights, deep dish pizza in Marquette Park, jazz at home, tea time, riding the el, climbing, Harper Library, LPs." After several rounds, they are smiling. After a few more, they begin to laugh. Even Melissa begins to feel light, and easy.

After several rounds, John says, "Leaving home."

Doug interjects, "Leaving here."

They close in tacit consensus. Their meals come. They eat in near silence for a while and then return to chitchat with long, comfortable pauses. Afterwards, as they walk down 53rd Street, Melissa watches John and realizes that when the difficult decision of the day is behind them, she will not need to lean on him anymore. Her love for him, though sometimes salty, is free of sorrow, and the challenges that they are facing together are slowly and steadily preparing them for joy.

"I love you all," Melissa says. She expects Doug to mock her for being mushy, or Sarah to probe her meaning with precise love words like philos, and metta, and agape, but neither replies. *They are glad to be loved.* Melissa feels a strange joy akin to hope and to the love she has for her patients. "Someday, I will love everything we shared here. But for now, I love all of you, and April and Alan too, more than I can say."

Epilogue

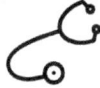

"It's 2020. We should see everything clearly now."

"For instance?"

"How we got into this mess and stayed in it."

"You're too hard-working and I'm too loyal. Or maybe this is exactly what was supposed to happen."

"You mean this was as good an outcome as we could have expected?"

"Yes. And a wonderful view."

"I can believe in you, and in the Finger Lakes?"

"And I can believe in you, and our work."

"That is a happy ending."

Melissa and John are sitting on the deck behind Sarah's sister's farm, watching the sun set over Lake Cayuga. The air is fresh and clear and the sun gentle; they have a few more minutes alone together, as the mist gathers, before they go inside to dine with Sarah, Doug, April, Alan, Randall, and a house full of other guests from near and far. They are older now, and though their bond is as strong as ever, it is easier to enjoy it while fully clothed.

"Your fertility and restoration clinic in the Amanas sounds wonderful."

"You're welcome to come and visit sometime. I really enjoyed seeing yours in Ithaca. It's just what I had hoped it might be—and more inspiring than I expected."

"It's our brainchild. We've been using your self-patterning for discovery for several years now, and the ripple effects are spreading."

"It gives me chills to hear that. Thank you. I had hoped that we might, um, give birth to my dream of a residential habitat restoration clinic and community."

"We did—you and I have the clinics and Randall and Sarah have the community."

"Who'd'a thunk it? Randall's community is living our dream, and Sarah's a part of it!"

"We've been expressing our fertility with each other through our dearest and oldest friends. We probably couldn't have done that in the old way."

"I agree. We share a lifework and legacy of great purpose and meaning. We're very lucky."

"You think so? You don't regret being sick? Or the consequences?"

"Forgetfulness and numbness are small prices to pay for the feeling that I did all I could to catalyze the survival of our species as the body of life."

"As Galileo put it, we had the chance—and took it—to be pilgrim minds."

"And, like those who started the modern era after the black death, to learn from our plagues how to make a new and better era."

Melissa stands and reaches out her hand. John takes it. They walk hand-in-hand up the bank through the twilight to the Chinese lanterns and warm laughter of the gathering in and around the old Quaker homestead.

Acknowledgments

For spiritual teachings that informed the development of the characters as they are in this book, I am grateful to: Rabbi Ted Falcon, Imam Jamal Rachman, Rodney Smith, Eight Limbs Yoga, Seattle Yoga Arts, Shoshone *ashram*, and the community of Bastyr University. I am also indebted to the light and dark education offered by the University of Chicago and its neighborhood and city, and to Valois's cafe and the small business community of Hyde Park and Kenwood.

For articulating and disseminating methods that provide a fast track to new knowledge when one is desperately needed, I as a late modern with the burning questions depicted in this novel owe my new and better life—my emerging cure—to: Berton Roueché, whose medical detective stories inspired me to specialize in Preventive Medicine and Public Health; William H. McNeill, whose *Plagues and Peoples* linked human history with medical history; Drs. David Sackett and Thomas Chalmers for championing the N-of-1 study and other applications in medicine of the long narrative case study; to Hope Jahren for doing the same for lab girls; and to A. R. Luria and Oliver Sacks for doing so in neurology.

For making it seem natural for a woman of my generation to enter medicine, I thank those who went before, especially Drs.

Kate Dobson, Peggy Telfer, and Elaine Hambrick. For showing what it takes to "leave the herd" and discover the new in medicine, I am grateful to Semmelweis, Dr. Carlos Findlay, Dr. Howard Taylor Ricketts, and Drs. Barry Marshall and Robin Warren. For keeping big-picture biological thinking alive in the era of reductionism, I am eternally grateful to Rachel Carson, Elizabeth Kolbert, Levins and Lewontin, and Charles Mann. For giving the teaching anecdote new life, I thank Dr. Rachel Naomi Riven.

I am grateful to the Southern Oregon team that made this book beautiful. The appearance is due to the professional competence and creativity of cover artist Bruce Bayard and book designer Chris Molé. The readability is due mainly to coach Chansonette Buck and editors Deidre Krupp, Deborah Mokma, and Ann DiSalvo.

Such writing ability as I am developing, I owe first to my father, who taught me reading and writing at a young age. I am also grateful to editor friends Eva Silverfine and Stephanie Holt for their talent and skill in verbal expression, to writing teachers Andrea Goldsmith of the Victorian Writer's Centre, and to Wendy Call of Hugo House. They kindly put up with an unusual and neurotoxic student, trusting that their wisdom would not go to waste.

Thank you also to my book development and beta readers, especially: Jan Agosti, Anna Barón, Jessica Bondy, Cynthia Bradley, Julie Clayton, Stephanie Holt, Christopher Howell, Joel Mason, Sara Myers Wade, Berta Nicol-Blades, and Dana Smaller. Special thanks to Jan, Anna, Julie, and Stephanie for their kindness in dark times.

About the Author

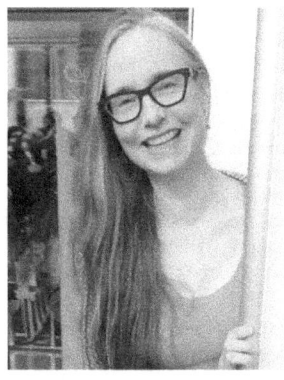

Beth Alderman, MD, MPH earned her AB and MD degrees from the University of Chicago and her MPH from the University of Washington. After Board Certification in Preventive Medicine and Public Health, she took a faculty position in the University of Colorado Medical School Department of Preventive Medicine, Biometrics, and Medical Informatics, where she did population-based epidemiological studies of adverse reproductive outcomes and methodological studies in clinical epidemiology. In her next faculty position at the University of Washington School of Public Health, she focused on risk factors for birth defects.

In 1996, she fell ill with the mysterious new plague and was given the provisional diagnosis "chronic fatigue syndrome". She has spent her time since studying her own case and pondering the reasons that her beloved profession failed her so completely. Fortunately, she discovered her cure, which may be of use to others suffering from one or more of the emerging epidemics affecting humans, their habitats, and life on earth.

For more about and from the author, see the following websites:

BethAldermanMD.com	*Free Information for all readers*
DoctorsOfLife.com	*For care and cure of all lives as one*
LivingFutureBooks.com	*Publishing Website*
LivingFutureCourses.com	*Educational Website with Free and advanced Courses*

Look for author's books on Amazon.com

Other Books by
Beth Alderman

Medical Phenomenology:
Chronic Ambient Poisoning

ISBN: 978-1-7332849-2-9

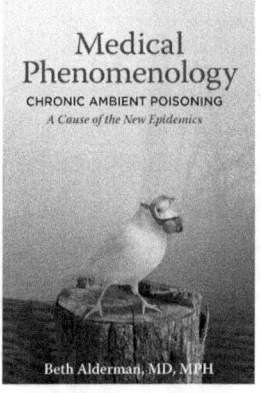

One day in December of 1996, the author (a physician, medical detective, and academic epidemiologist) developed disabling brain fog following on a decade-long descent into a painful, pervasive, and unprecedented chronic illness. Having done population-based studies to research the causes of birth defects, and having thus encountered the limitations of modern methods, she had inadvertently prepared to investigate the causes of her illness—which was given the provisional and uninformative label of "chronic fatigue."

The author began a delineation of the natural history of her condition using the methods of: doctors Hippocrates, Maimonides and Oliver Sacks; the "radical empiricism" used by Dr. William James; and the phenomenology introduced by Teilhard de Chardin and Merleau-Ponty. After a fifteen-year search, she found a doctor of integrative medicine whose elimination diet relieved her brain fog, which enabled her to complete a self-study and to construct an actionable new diagnosis: chronic ambient poisoning. Unseen by doctors and obscured by medical dogma and a myriad of false diagnoses, chronic ambient poisoning defies late modern, fragmented, accuracy-challenged medical research methods and delivery systems. It also reveals that human-caused habitat injuries that afflict birds, bees, and other species are affecting humans while driving evolved life toward extinction in the way of an asteroid strike. To ignore this diagnosis is to ignore the dangers to all lives posed by maladaptive modern lifeways.

The Evolve Fertility Series

BOOK 1
Melissa's Match: *Great Society*
ISBN: 978-1-7321110-1-1

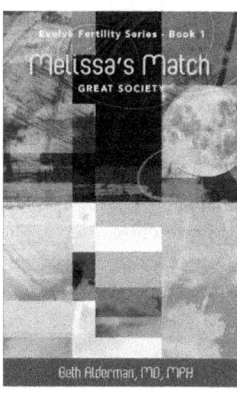

It's the early 1970s. Melissa and her friends begin their first year of college in the inner city of Chicago at a time when post-assassination riots, Great Society scholarship programs, and veterans returning from Vietnam create a sometimes explosive confluence of urban and rural, rich and poor, white and black, educated and uneducated. Coming of age in a violent, unjust, and yet hopeful time, they struggle to reconcile their hopes and opportunities with the shadows of war and the destructive clashes of senescing and emerging systems of care and cure of life on earth.

BOOK 2
Connie's Conception: *Awareness of Peril*
ISBN: 978-1-7321110-0-4

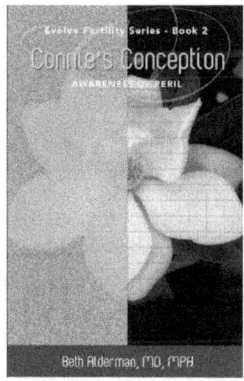

It's the late 1980s, and Connie Martin, a doctor working for the Epidemiology Intelligence Service of the CDC, is called to Colorado to investigate an alarming outbreak of birth defects. Born illegitimate in the San Luis Valley as Consuela Martín, a name known only to close friends and to her beloved gamer and programmer husband, she arrives as an unknown. Joined by environmental activists who suspect the state's Superfund sites and by doctors and parents who fear for its children, Connie attempts to discover the link between habitat destruction and damage to innocents.

BOOK 3
Melissa's Malady: *End of Modernity*
ISBN: 978-1-7321110-2-8

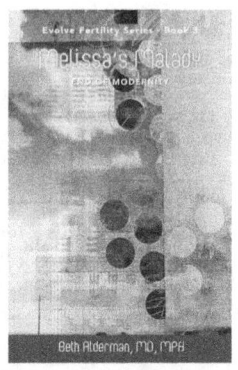

IIt is almost the year of the millennium, and Melissa meets her college friends Sarah and Doug and her first and only true love John for a reunion in Hyde Park. All four are in the midst of their careers. All struggle with the compromises that have marred their happiness. All wish to change the world, each in a different way. Sarah has left her government job for a new life as a yoga teacher. Doug is helping to birth a new value-based economy. John is a successful academic doctor. Melissa is ailing. They unite to turn John's success as a researcher to the cure of Melissa's mysterious chronic illness. What they find will change their lives and their imperiled world.

BOOK 4
Colette's Creativity: *Sacred and Profane*
ISBN: 978-1-7321110-3-5

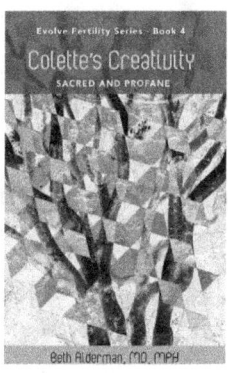

Colette, Melissa's childhood friend, abandons her marriage and home in Maine and flies to Melbourne. There she is taken in by her friend Reggie, who seems to know the secret of joy. Colette joins in the lives of striking individuals who lead her to view sexuality as a manifestation of the sacred. As she leaves behind the wounds caused by profane sexuality, she and her new friends clash with members of Reggie's family who force them to flee and to begin again.

BOOK 5
Colette's Community: *Thirds*
ISBN: 978-1-7321110-4-2

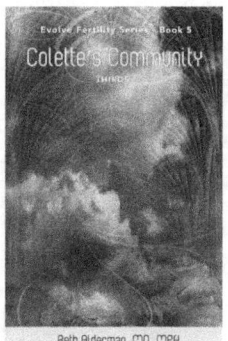

Soon after Colette and her friends find a new home, an old boyfriend of Melissa's who is sojourning in Australia calls and expresses his desire to visit. Colette plans to use the visit as a chance to develop a job for herself; he plans to check up on Colette for Melissa. As they get to know each other, they see that despite differences in religion, origin, and experience, they are on very similar spiritual paths. When it is time for Randall to go home, Colette joins him in Chicago. When he becomes caught up in his old life, however, she returns to Australia to pursue her dream of giving birth to a sacred community.

Chronic Illness Owner's Manuals

Regenerate Your Life: Chronic Illness as a Springboard for Creating Your Best Life

ISBN: 978-1-7321110-8-0 (VOL. 1)

ISBN: 978-1-7321110-9-7 (VOL. 2)

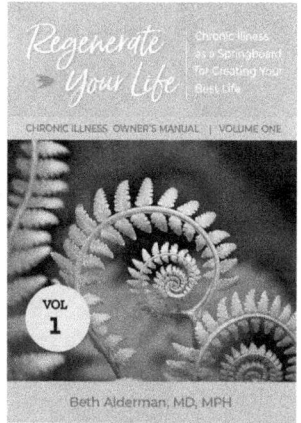

The *Chronic Illness Owner's Manual* series is for patients with chronic illness, and for the people who care for them. Suitable for individual or small group use, it offers a comprehensive, systematic, step-by-step approach to engaging modern medical systems, and to healing from the inside out.

The books comprise anecdotes, exercises, and quotes that address recovery through seven aspects of the body: awareness, understanding, perceptions, sensations, energy, flesh, and interbeing. The frames, constructs, patterns, and processes employed by the series are drawn from traditions of medicine, field biology, theology, and psychology from around the globe. Their synthesis offers an emerging, sustainable, eco-centric, eco-contextual, and customizable approach to creating a new and better life that regenerates your unique meaning, purpose, and vision of abundant life. The *Chronic Illness Owner's Manual* series complements care and cure courses available online at www. LivingFutureCourses.com.

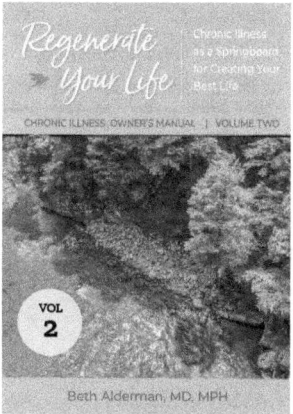

The Evolve Restoration Series
Sequel to the Evolve Fertility Series

BOOK 1
Pilgrim Minds: *After the War on Life*
ISBN: 978-1-7321110-5-9

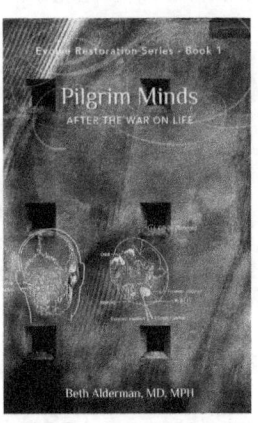

Melissa's deathbed request catapults her son Aaron on a journey from her family's Mississippian clinic to the Salish Sea to claim a mysterious legacy. Meeting his niece Rafa en route, he continues overland with her, and uncle and niece come to know and depend on each other. On arriving at the Saltspring Island Research Center (SIRC), Sarah, now the keeper of the center's narratives, confesses that Aaron's legacy is a task: to apply his mother's philosophy to SIRC's lifeways in order to revitalize it.

While he had been immersed in his mother's medical philosophy, SIRC had used many of her ideas to found a fertility school. SIRC's encroaching apathy persuaded Sarah that they missed one or more essential lifeways, and hopes that Aaron may be able to pinpoint and provide them. Taken by surprise, but ready to step up, Aaron immerses himself in the community, and Rafa undergoes SIRC's initiation process. Uncle and niece come to love Cascadia and to relish local, burgeoning patterns of innovation. Both choose to stay at SIRC, an agentic community that is doing much to restore evolution and its living future.

BOOK 2
Aaron's Legacy: *The Body of Life*
ISBN: 978-1-7321110-6-6

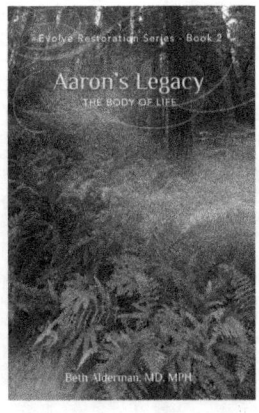

Having come to know the community, Aaron receives his legacy as a series of enactments of SIRC's history. The surviving members of his mother's old friendship group—Sarah, Doug, and John—join the audience and performers in processing and adapting their shared narrative. In the intervals between enactments, Rafa undergoes initiation while Aaron explores the composer, an instrument that enables a player to evoke memories with images and to express the player's responses as sound scapes. As Aaron shares his with Rafa, Sarah and others, John shares memories of Melissa, and seems to receive a new message from her.

As the community adapts to changes in its meaning and purpose, Rafa and Aaron each finds a first consort and draws inspiration from local knowledge keepers and change agents residing at SIRC, the nearby Monastery of Origins and Endings, or in Victoria or Vancouver. Aaron's health, damaged by his travel through a poison barren, deteriorates. With his death, his consort Parvati shares their legacy in the form of patterns of action that may remove roadblocks to continuous adaptation and renewal.

BOOK 3

The Kindred's Rebirth: *Rough Seas and Far Lands*

ISBN: 978-1-7332849-3-6

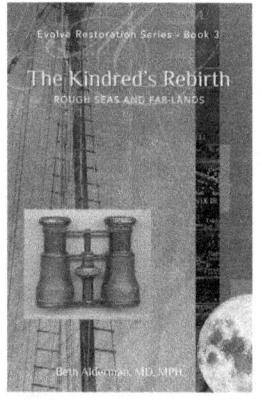

A decade later in Australia, Parvati and Björn give up on effecting meaningful restoration there. Dirk, while on his annual circuit of the north, arrives in Jokkmokk for the annual Sámi gathering to learn that SIRC is in crisis. Rafa, who is crossing the South Pacific on her two year global clinic circuit, hears strange news: the Fertility School, which was winding down, closed without notice. She realizes that her work, too, is drawing to a close as her clinics adapt to localism and begin to diverge.

All three travelers feel a strong homing urge and hatch a plan to converge in Scandinavia with the remnant of the SIRC community. En route, Parvati adopts a grandchild, Jacki, who helps Björn to recover from a disorder of interbeing. Many new consort pairs join the kindred and revive it by helping to form a next community, SIRC-Umea, and to organize and maintain residential restoration communities in the Baltic and North Sea bioregions, and to recover from the painful loss of the original community.

BOOK 4

Jacki's Vision: *The Green Line*

ISBN: 978-1-7332849-4-3

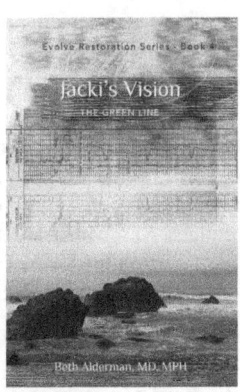

When Jacki turns sixteen, she begins her transition to adulthood by venturing into larger worlds of knowledge and adaptation to gain skills. During her first clinic circuit in the Baltic, she finds that her coming of age is coinciding with her kindred's restiveness. As she embraces and contemplates her future, a vision takes hold of her. She proposes a Green Line restoration project in Tasmania to reconcile a time debt created by the Black Line genocide, and to prepare her for organizing bioregional restoration projects. Her kindred and their networks embrace the project, expand it, and multiply its potential effects.

As the Green Line Corps prepares to depart en masse for Tasmania, Jacki meets a young stranger, Mirek, whose experience of the world—whose very umwelt—contrasts with her own. Later, in Tasmania, she gains a consort, Izaak, and a sister friend, Lally, both of whom winnow her possible futures. Together, the many thousands of Green Line participants develop a restoration ethos and synchronize living processes for restoring habitats—with their restorers. Jacki and her new peers are among the first to return to the original SIRC campus, near which many former kindred members have settled, and to which many others are about to return.

BOOK 5

Mel's Motherhood: *A Place in the Living World*

ISBN: 978-1-7332849-5-0

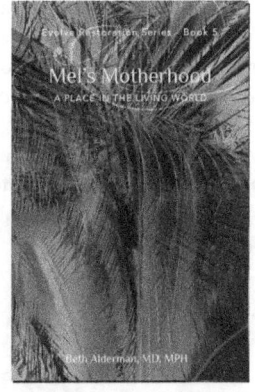

Mel and JJ—children of the Three Mammas—await the advance boat from Tasmania at the Cascadian Monastery of Origins and Endings. Mel, who is pregnant, and JJ, who fared poorly while he was away, finished their initiation projects and are keen to see Jacki and to meet the new kindred members. In the course of a joyful reunion, Mel and JJ learn that Jacki and Lally are also pregnant.

As this next generation of adults chooses ways to express fertility and defines new vocations, the reconstituting kindred celebrates new human lives, integrates with local communities, and processes hitherto hidden threads of SIRC's history with the aid of DNA fathers who participate. The complex, complementary communities adapt to continuous learning via phenomenology, and to continuous adaptation of systems for care and cure of evolved life.

Meaningful Retirement: *Become a Life Care Provider*

ISBN: 978-1-7332849-0-5

Meaningful Retirement is a self-guided monthly course in four seasons that can aid people like you who are exiting modern employment or withdrawing from the modern death economy. In it you will find a toolbox for transition to a vocation of life care, and thus begin to mature into a wise elder able to lead and mentor those who follow you. These seasons include:

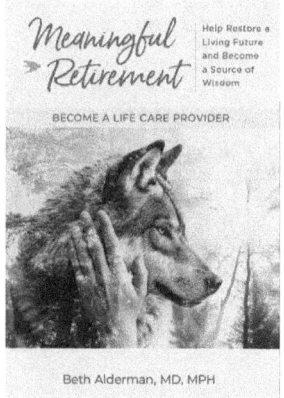

- **A Summer Breather**
- **A Fall for Reflection**
- **A Winter to Reclaim Your Personal Narrative**
- **A Spring for Revolutionizing Your Lifetime Learning**

As you transition to the role of provider of life care, you may choose to co-found emotionally and spiritually astute communities where you can mentor your juniors, who face the imminent and daunting task of passing through wrenching psycho-social change while arresting and reversing the accelerating human-caused Sixth Extinction. That threat to evolved life represents a unique crucible for transforming modern lifeways into ones that enable humans to choose and to restore life. Re-visioning and co-creating processes of care and cure that restore all lives as one will prepare your species to restore the planet's living lungs, its water circulation, its living shade, and its evolved resilience to unexpected planetary catastrophes. By viewing life in time though an eco-centric and eco-contextualized lens that scales from your lifetime to evolutionary time, you can begin to see your world through new eyes that reveal your place in the big picture of life on earth.

Direct learning, that is, phenomenology, is essential for restoration of a living future. This method has changed with every epoch since ancient natural historians began to attempt to create views, frames, and constructs in an attempt to grasp evolving generative systems. The present moment of peril can be taken as an impetus and inspiration to engage with an exciting process of learning and problem solving that some call the living paradigm. This paradigm, which is still incubating in fields as diverse as architecture and design, agriculture, archaeology, restoration, and theology, is ripe for grass roots syncreses across outdated fields of knowledge. When you learn to cooperate with the last hundreds of millions of years of evolution while pursuing space age ways of averting asteroid collision, you will be prepared to lead your species toward sustainability and to make room for rapid human adaptation that restores evolution. Welcome to the One Life..

www.ingramcontent.com/pod-product-compliance
Lightning Source LLC
Chambersburg PA
CBHW070000200626
46811CB00021B/2815